D1071653

Noninvasive Brain Imaging:

Computed Tomography and Radionuclides

Noninvasive Brain Imaging:

Computed Tomography and Radionuclides

Edited by

Harold J. DeBlanc, Jr., M.D.
Director, Nuclear Medicine
University of Utah

James A. Sorenson, Ph.D.
Director, Medical Physics
University of Utah

Published by THE SOCIETY OF NUCLEAR MEDICINE, INC., NEW YORK, N.Y.

Distributed by PUBLISHING SCIENCES GROUP, INC., ACTON, MASS.

Distributed by
   Publishing Sciences Group, Inc.
   162 Great Road
   Acton, Massachusetts 01720

ISBN 0-88416-137-4

This volume is affectionately dedicated to
Georgie
and
Lucy

Participants

Philip Braunstein
New York University Medical Center
New York, New York

Thomas F. Budinger
University of California
Berkeley, California

R. Edward Coleman
Washington University School of
  Medicine
Mallinkrodt Institute of Radiology
St. Louis, Missouri

Ernest W. Fordham
Rush-Presbyterian,
  St. Luke's Medical Center
Chicago, Illinois

John C. Harbert
Georgetown University Medical Center
Washington, D.C.

Paul B. Hoffer
University of California, San Francisco
San Francisco, California

David E. Kuhl
Hospital of the University of Pennsylvania
Philadelphia, Pennsylvania

William H. Oldendorf
University of California
School of Medicine
Los Angeles, California

Anthony M. Passalaqua
New York University Medical Center
New York, New York

Michael E. Phelps
Washington University School of
  Medicine
Mallinckrodt Institute of Radiology
St. Louis, Missouri

Henry N. Wagner, Jr.
The Johns Hopkins Medical Institutions
Baltimore, Maryland

Michael J. Welch
Washington University School of
  Medicine
Mallinckrodt Institute of Radiology
St. Louis, Missouri

Contributors

Abass Alavi
Hospital of the University of Pennsylvania
Philadelphia, Pennsylvania

Philip O. Alderson
Washington University School of
  Medicine
Mallinckrodt Institute of Radiology
St. Louis, Missouri

Stewart P. Axelbaum
Georgetown University Medical Center
Washington, D.C.

John J. Bouz
Foothills Hospital
Calgary, Alberta, Canada

Norman E. Chase
New York University Medical Center
New York, New York

Frank H. DeLand
University of Kentucky Medical Center
Lexington, Kentucky

Giovanni DiChiro
NINDS, National Institutes of Health
Washington, D.C.

Hector E. Duggan
Foothills Hospital
Calgary, Alberta, Canada

Roy Q. Edwards
Hospital of the University of Pennsylvania
Philadelphia, Pennsylvania

John O. Eichling
Washington University School of
  Medicine
Mallinckrodt Institute of Radiology
St. Louis, Missouri

Craig A. Fenton
Hospital of the University of Pennsylvania
Philadelphia, Pennsylvania

Mokhtar Gado
Washington University School of
  Medicine
Mallinckrodt Institute of Radiology
St. Louis, Missouri

Randolph O. George
The Johns Hopkins Medical Institutions
Baltimore, Maryland

Edward J. Hoffman
Washington University School of
  Medicine
Mallinckrodt Institute of Radiology
St. Louis, Missouri

Bernard Hoop, Jr.
Massachusetts General Hospital
Boston, Massachusetts

Irvin I. Kricheff
New York University Medical Center
New York, New York

William T. McLaughlin
Santa Clara Valley Medical Center
San Jose, California

Nizar A. Mullani
Washington University School of Medicine
St. Louis, Missouri

Thomas P. Naidich
New York University Medical Center
New York, New York

Marcus E. Raichle
Washington University School of
  Medicine
Mallinckrodt Institute of Radiology
St. Louis, Missouri

Martin M. Reivich
Hospital of the University of Pennsylvania
Philadelphia, Pennsylvania

Dieter Schellinger
Georgetown University Medical Center
Washington, D.C.

Maria G. Straatmann
Washington University School of
  Medicine
Mallinckrodt Institute of Radiology
St. Louis, Missouri

Michel M. Ter-Pogossian
Washington University School of
  Medicine
Mallinckrodt Institute of Radiology
St. Louis, Missouri

David A. Turner
Rush-Presbyterian,
  St. Luke's Medical Center
Chicago, Illinois

Paul M. Weber
Kaiser-Permanente Medical Center
Oakland, California

Robert A. Zimmerman
Hospital of the University of Pennsylvania
Philadelphia, Pennsylvania

Contents

Foreword

For the past 10 years radionuclide imaging of the brain has provided a reliable and useful technique for the diagnosis of brain disease. The low cost and noninvasive nature of the procedure has made it the screening test of choice for brain disease. The role of radionuclide brain imaging has recently been challenged, however, by the development of a new transmission scanning technique, computerized transaxial tomography, or CTT scanning.

Seldom has a new diagnostic technique received such rapid acceptance as CTT scanning. It has been suggested that this may have a profound impact on the routine use of radionuclide brain imaging. It is therefore desirable at this time to examine the roles of these two techniques in the diagnosis of brain disease and to evaluate the potential for future developments. This book presents such an assessment by several leading experts in the field.

The first two chapters are devoted to the present status of radionuclide brain imaging and to current concepts of the blood-brain barrier and its importance in radionuclide studies, particularly in regard to the development of new radiopharmaceuticals for brain imaging. The next five chapters discuss other new concepts and potential future developments. These include the use of new radiopharmaceuticals, especially those containing cyclotron-produced radionuclides, including ^{11}C, ^{13}N, and ^{15}O. The desirable decay characteristics of these radionuclides and their importance as labels for physiological compounds have long been recognized. The technology for labeling these compounds has been demonstrated. What remains to be done is to develop relatively inexpensive methods for producing them in a clinical environment. It should be noted that the cost of the currently available compact cyclotron even now is not too different from that of a single CTT scanner, and there is potential for the development of a lower cost, smaller, medical cyclotron more suitable for routine clinical use.

Computerized reconstruction tomography in brain imaging is not, of course, new or unique to transmission techniques since it was introduced by Kuhl and coworkers in nuclear medicine over 10 years ago. The work of these investigators in the development of computerized radionuclide transaxial tomography, or CRTT scanning, summarized in Chapter 5, is particularly worthy of review at this time. Also presented in other chapters are descriptions of techniques and early clinical results for reconstruction tomography employing the scintillation camera and a new imaging device for positron emitters. The latter is of particular importance with respect to the cyclotron-produced radionuclides mentioned earlier. It is possible that, by providing improved images and new tests using new radiopharmaceuticals, CRTT imaging could have as great an impact as CTT scanning on the diagnosis of brain disease.

The last five chapters are devoted to CTT and radionuclide scanning, including comparisons of clinical results obtained by both procedures. Chapter 8 presents an especially useful and comprehensive analysis of the capabilities and limitations of current CTT scanners as well as a discussion of their potential for further improvements. The final chapter presents a panel discussion among a variety of experts in radionuclide and CTT scanning.

It is expected that other noninvasive brain-imaging techniques besides those discussed here may also be developed further in the next few years. One of these, for example, is the use of improved diagnostic ultrasound techniques. While their potential is recognized, however, a discussion of these techniques was considered beyond the scope of this book.

We are grateful to Dr. Monte Blau for his support and assistance in the careful review of this work and to Margaret Glos and Christa Foster of the Society of Nuclear Medicine for their help in the organization of the symposium given in Salt Lake City and for their continued assistance throughout the publication of this volume. We are also indebted to Margaret Ann Bowman for her patient and diligent performance in the extensive task of preparing the typewritten manuscripts. Finally, we would like to thank the authors for their promptness in reviewing and returning the edited manuscripts, which helped to make rapid publication of this book possible.

HAROLD J. DeBLANC, JR.
JAMES A. SORENSON

Chapter 1

Ten Years of Brain Tumor Scanning at Johns Hopkins: 1962–1972

Randolph O. George and Henry N. Wagner, Jr.

The enormous technological advances that we are observing today in the fields of diagnostic radiology and nuclear medicine, particularly in relation to the study of brain disease, suggest that it may be worthwhile to review our past experience to gain insight into possible future developments. In this chapter we will review our experiences in brain tumor scanning over the past 10 years at the Johns Hopkins Hospital. Included in our discussion will be changes in technology that have occurred, the relationship of brain scanning to other diagnostic procedures in patients with neurological disease, the sensitivity of brain scanning for the detection of tumors, the effect of various diagnostic procedures on the interval between onset of symptoms and time of surgery for brain tumors, and changes in the operative mortality and 2-year survival of patients with a variety of brain tumors.

Materials and Methods

During the period from January 1, 1962, to May 1, 1972, 1,050 patients with the diagnosis of "brain tumor" were seen at the Johns Hopkins Hospital. The subjects selected for this study included only those among this group meeting the following additional criteria: (A) intracranial brain tumor confirmed by tissue diagnosis; (B) brain scans performed within 1 year preceding the diagnosis; and (C) all other neurological procedures performed at the Johns Hopkins Hospital. Of the 1,050 patients, 369 (35%) met all of the criteria prescribed for inclusion in this study.

The relative sensitivities of brain scans, arteriograms, and air studies for all tumors were examined with regard to tumor location and type of tumor. Types of tumor were divided into four groups: meningiomas, astrocytomas, metastases, and all tumors. We also investigated the relationship between scan positivity and the number of months the scan was performed after the onset of symptoms.

Brain-scanning techniques underwent progressive change at our institution over the 10-year period. Figure 1-1 shows one of the earliest brain scans performed at the Johns Hopkins Hospital. The scan is a lateral view obtained with a rectilinear scanner with a 3-in.-diam NaI(Tl) detector 24 hr after injection of ^{131}I-labeled serum albumin. The use of ^{99m}Tc-pertechnetate began in 1964. Initially, a 10-mCi dose was injected intravenously without perchlorate or atropine, and anterior, posterior, and two lateral scan views were obtained. Since 1966, atropine and potassium perchlorate have been added to the protocol and the dose has progressively increased to its current level of 15–20 mCi. Vertex views were obtained routinely after the mid-1960s. Use of the Anger camera began in 1967 and has progressively increased (Fig. 1-2) until at this time the camera and scanner are used with about equal frequency. More recently, computer analysis has been added (1), and in many cases cerebral circula-

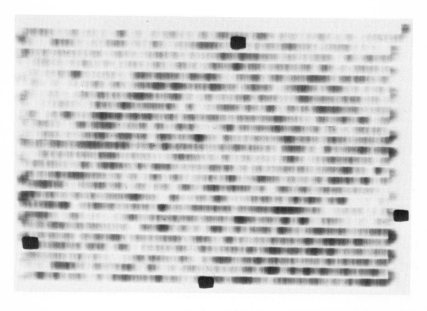

Fig. 1-1. One of earliest brain scans at Johns Hopkins Medical Institutions performed with rectilinear scanner with 3-in.-diam NaI(Tl) crystal after injection of ^{131}I-labeled serum albumin.

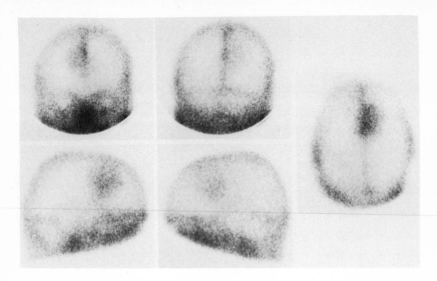

Fig. 1-2. Routine five-view brain scan of patient with meningioma performed with Anger camera and 15 mCi ^{99m}Tc-pertechnetate.

tion is evaluated from serial camera images obtained 2 sec apart after intravenous injection of the tracer as bolus (2) (Fig. 1-3).

Results

Frequency of studies. The number of brain scans increased by nearly a factor of 10 over the decade 1962–1972 (Fig. 1-4). From 1965 on, the number of arteriograms increased parallel with the number of scans, although the latter was about three times more numerous. By contrast, the number of air studies appeared to decrease slightly.

Relative accuracy. As shown in Fig. 1-5, the percentage of true positive brain scans did not change significantly over the 10-year period, remaining about 77% for all tumor types despite improvements in scanning techniques. Our accuracy level of 77% is somewhat lower than those of other reported series (3–5), which range between 82% and 84%, and equal to that reported by Wang, et al (6). The reasons for these differences are unknown.

Table 1-1 summarizes the number and percentage of positive pertechnetate scans and compares these to results of cerebral angiography, electroencephalography (EEG), and air studies (Air) for tumor type. For EEG, a positive result was indicated by the presence of an electrical abnormality in the hemisphere where the tumor was located, while positive results for all other studies refer to precise tumor localization.

The overall accuracy of air contrast studies (89%) exceeded that

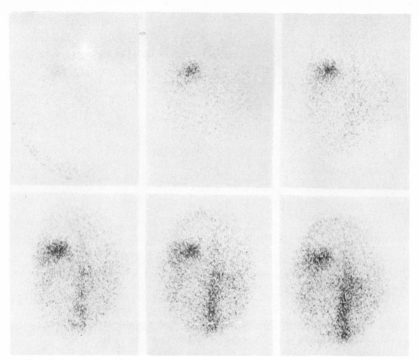

Fig. 1-3. Cerebral bloodflow study of patient with arteriovenous malformation.

of arteriography (84%), brain scanning (77%), and EEG (66%). However, air contrast studies were generally performed for the delineation of tumors in regions of the brain that are notoriously difficult to study by arteriography and brain scanning. The high detection rate by air studies of tumors near the posterior fossa and brain stem probably contributes significantly to the overall high percentage of positive air studies.

Accuracy as a function of location. Table 1-2 summarizes the accuracy of scanning, angiography, and air studies in relation to location of the tumor. Frontal tumors were detected more frequently by arteriography (82%) than by scans (77%) or air studies (70%). Parasagittal tumors were detected with greater than 93% accuracy by all three types of studies. Arteriograms detected 100% of temporal tumors, compared to 83% for air studies and 81% for scans. There was little difference in detection rate of parietal tumors (89–94%) among the three types of studies. Scans and arteriograms were similarly effective (90% and 86%) for detection of occipital tumors. There were no air studies in this group. Thalamic, sellar, and parasellar tumors were more accurately detected by air studies (92%) than by arteriograms (84%) or scans (60%). Both scans and arteriograms de-

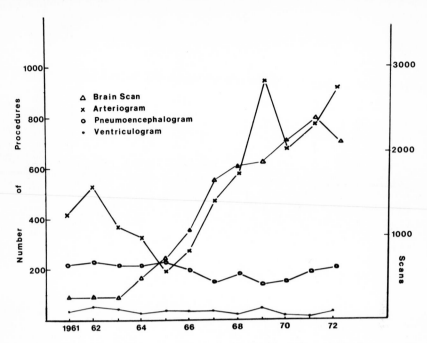

Fig. 1-4. Comparison of numbers of radiographic studies and brain scans performed.

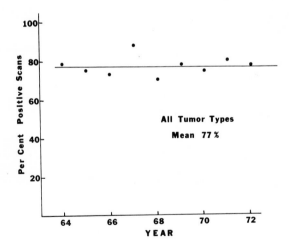

Fig. 1-5. Percentage of positive scans in all tumor types over the decade.

tected 100% of sphenoid wing meningiomas. These were not studied with air contrast procedures. Pontine tumors were most effectively detected by air studies and arteriography (78% and 80%), and least often by scanning (25%), the lowest scanning detection rate for any

TABLE 1-1. Proven Brain Tumors Studied with Pertechnetate Brain Scans, Cerebral Angiography, Electroencephalography, and Air Studies

Diagnosis	No. patients	Scan		Angiogram		EEG		Air	
		Positive Total	= %	Positive Total	= %	Positive Total	= %	Positive Total	= %
Astrocytoma	101	89/121	74	94/104	90	64/84	76	43/46	93
Meningioma	91	100/107	93	91/99	92	38/59	64	15/17	88
Metastatic	67	59/80	74	38/51	75	28/41	68	11/17	65
Pituitary adenoma	22	15/23	65	18/21	86	2/8	25	12/13	92
Acoustic neuroma	13	13/14	93	4/10	40	2/6	33	1/2	50
Craniopharyngioma	12	4/15	27	12/15	80	5/9	56	10/10	100
Ependymoma	11	8/12	67	6/10	60	4/8	50	7/8	88
Medulloblastoma	7	5/9	56	4/6	67	5/7	71	6/6	100
Optic glioma	4	2/4	50	1/2	50	—	—	1/1	100
Miscellaneous	4	3/4	75	1/4	25	2/4	50	1/1	100
Angioblastoma	3	1/3	33	2/3	67	—	—	—	—
Oligodendroglioma	2	3/3	100	3/3	100	2/2	100	—	—
Total	337	302/395	76.5	274/328	83.5	152/229	66.4	107/121	88.4

TABLE 1-2. Accuracy of Scanning, Angiography, and Air Studies in Relation to Location

Location	Scan		Angiogram		Air	
	Positive/Total	= %	Positive/Total	= %	Positive/Total	= %
Frontal	68/88	77	53/65	82	14/20	70
Frontoparietal or parasagittal	35/36	97	26/28	93	5/5	100
Temporal	30/37	81	31/31	100	5/6	83
Parietal	68/75	91	56/63	89	15/16	94
Occipital	9/10	90	6/7	86	—	
Thalamic, sellar, or parasellar	45/75	60	58/69	84	34/37	92
Sphenoid wing	14/14	100	14/14	100	—	
Pons	3/12	25	7/9	78	5/6	83
Cerebellopontine angle	19/20	95	8/14	57	4/5	80
Medulla or cerebellum	26/49	53	18/34	53	31/34	91
Total	317/416	76	277/334	83	113/129	88

anatomic region. Cerebellopontine-angle tumors, largely acoustic neuromas and meningiomas, were much more readily detected by scanning (95%) than by air studies (80%) or arteriography (57%). Medullary and cerebellar tumors were accurately found in 91% of air studies, compared to 53% of both scans and arteriograms.

In general, air contrast studies were most effective in detecting brain tumors whenever they were used, with the important qualifications that a predominance of paraventricular tumors were studied and many tumors were not studied at all with air. Arteriograms detected 85% and brain scans 76% of the total group. Brain scans were distinctly superior to other studies in detecting cerebellopontine-angle tumors (95%). Arteriograms were distinctly superior to other studies for frontal (81%) and temporal (100%) tumors. Scans and arteriograms were equally effective in detecting parietal, occipital, sphenoid, and posterior fossa tumors.

Relationship of accuracy to duration of symptoms. Approximately 93% of meningiomas were seen on scans performed at the onset of symptoms, and virtually all were detected after about 28 months of illness. About 67% of astrocytomas had positive scans at the onset of symptoms. A maximum detection rate of 87% was reached after about 28 months. Patients surviving beyond this time had slightly lower positive scanning results, possibly as a result of a lower grade of tumor malignancy or smaller-sized lesions.

Metastatic tumors were detected in about 67% of preoperative cases at the onset of symptoms, but scans became virtually 100% positive at 8 months, presumably related to rapid tumor growth. Metastases were associated with 100% positive scans throughout the 18 months after onset of symptoms. Patients surviving longer than 18 months showed a marked drop in scanning detection rate, probably as a result of a lower grade of tumor malignancy.

Correlation with surgery. Figure 1-6 illustrates that the number of operations for brain tumor increased only slightly from about 60 to 70 per year (this figure includes more than the basic 369 patients because all surgery patients were included). Figure 1-7 illustrates that the time between the onset of symptoms and the time of surgery decreased from as much as 4 years to less than 1 year.

Patient survival. Figure 1-8 shows an apparent increase in the 1-month survival after surgery for all types of brain tumors over the decade. However, this may be related to an improvement in the operative mortality. Despite the improvement in operative mortality, there was no apparent increase in survival 24 months after surgery (Fig. 1-9). This was true for all types of lesions, except possibly meningiomas, in which there was a slight improvement in survival from 60% to about 70%. Figure 1-10 illustrates the percent survival of

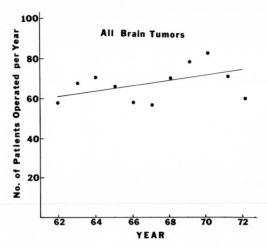

Fig. 1-6.   Number of patients who underwent surgery per year of all tumors.

patients with all types of tumors. It can be seen that there is no significant difference between the curves for 1963, 1966, 1969, and 1972.

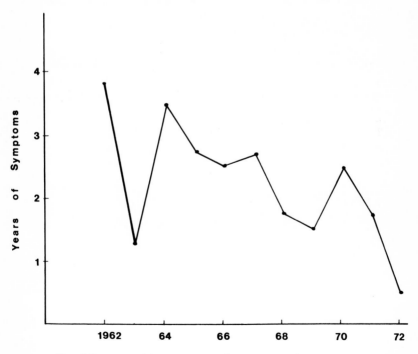

Fig. 1-7.   Interval between onset of symptoms and neurosurgery.

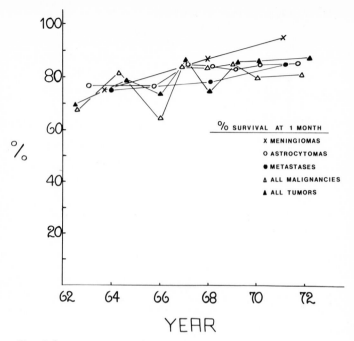

Fig. 1-8. Percent survival at 1 month after surgery of all tumors.

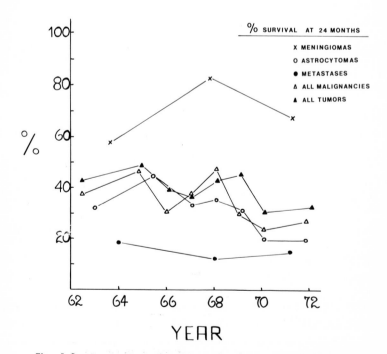

Fig. 1-9. Percent survival at 24 months after surgery of all tumors.

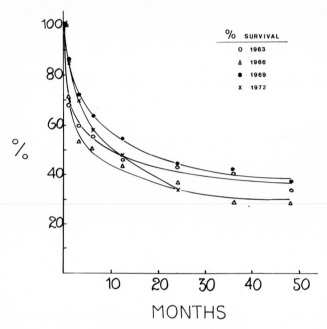

Fig. 1-10. Percent survival of all tumors.

Discussion

Some may feel a sense of disappointment at the results of this study. Although there was nearly a tenfold increase in the number of brain scans over the decade of the study, the number of patients with brain tumors who came to surgery did not increase significantly nor was there any apparent increase in 2-year survival. Harvey Cushing reported that for a series of 295 patients with intracranial meningiomas seen between 1927 and 1932, the overall operative mortality was 19.6% (7,8). Five-year mortality dropped from 18.4% to 12% over the period, most of which he attributed to the introduction of cryosurgery in 1927. He commented at the time that: "New methods will almost certainly have been introduced which in all likelihood will make our survival percentages for the final 1927–32 period by comparison appear to be amateurish and the work of tyros." Unfortunately, we do not seem to have done much better than Cushing, at least in terms of mortality.

However, as pointed out by Cushing in his book *Tumors of the Nervus Acusticus and the Syndrome of the Cerebellopontile Angle (9)*, first published in 1917, there are other important criteria in addition to the prolongation of life by which the success of neurosurgical procedures is judged. They include (A) the immediate or early operative fatalities, (B) postoperative complications, (C) degree of relief from suffering or avoidance of sequelae such as blindness, (D) capacity to renew former occupation, and (E) duration of the period of total or partial relief of symptoms.

These points suggest possible reasons why brain scanning has increased so dramatically over the past decade despite the apparent lack of effect on survival rates. Such reasons include the following:

1. Brain scanning helps to decrease morbidity. If patients with benign brain tumors such as meningiomas are operated on earlier, the loss of function of the brain and special senses, such as vision, is significantly less. In this regard, it is especially encouraging that the interval between the onset of symptoms and surgery decreased so dramatically over the decade of this study.
2. Brain scanning helps in making decisions about patients' problems. For example, it is important to know that a patient has a cerebral metastasis even though this knowledge will not improve his chances for survival. Such information is of value to the patient, to his family, and often to society, if, for example, the patient has an occupation such as an airplane pilot.
3. Brain scanning seems to have been most valuable for excluding the diagnosis of neurosurgical disease. For example, if a child has a focal seizure, a negative scan decreases the likelihood of a mass lesion to the point where the child can be treated with drugs and not require hospitalization for the more invasive procedures such as air contrast studies. Many patients who, in the past, would have been hospitalized and referred to neurosurgeons because of neurological symptoms can now be cared for by internists, pediatricians, and neurologists.
4. Brain scanning is performed not only for diagnosing brain tumors, but also for diagnosing cerebrovascular disease and infections. The ability to diagnose brain abscesses has been improved considerably since the introduction of brain scanning.

These considerations indicate a considerably greater value for brain scanning than is suggested by mortality data alone.

Summary

Between 1962 and 1972, 369 patients with proven intracranial tumors had brain scans at Johns Hopkins Hospital. The scan results were compared to those of cerebral angiography, air contrast studies, and electroencephalography. Scans were positive in 77% of cases; arteriograms, 83%; electroencephalograms, 66%; and air studies, 89%. Scanning was most effective for detecting meningiomas and acoustic neuromas. Angiograms were slightly more effective than scans for other tumors but were used less frequently because of the need for intra-arterial injection. Air studies were generally the most accurate diagnostic procedures for all except metastatic tumors. However, they were done selectively and were used much less frequently than the other procedures because of their technical requirements and potential for patient morbidity. Consistently low rates of tumor detection by brain scanning were seen in the brain stem and in the posterior fossa, with the notable exception of the cerebellopontine angle in which scanning results were superior to those of any of the other types of studies. All diagnostic procedures were similar (70–82% positive) in the frontal areas.

The various tumor types showed different degrees of uptake of ^{99m}Tc-pertechnetate over time. Metastatic tumors were seen most intensely from 8 to 18 months after onset of symptoms. Meningiomas and astrocytomas showed their greatest detection rate after 28 months of symptoms. This suggests that delayed scanning is often more effective than scanning soon after the onset of symptoms, and that serial scanning at periodic intervals may be useful.

The number of tumors that came to surgery and the survival 2 years after surgery did not increase greatly over the decade under study. The most important use of brain scanning seemed to be in making decisions about cerebrovascular disease, brain abscess, and brain tumor. Little effect on mortality from brain tumors was documented.

References

1. MOSES DC, NATARAJAN TK, PREZIOSI TJ: Quantitative cerebral circulation studies with sodium pertechnetate. *J Nucl Med* 14: 142–148, 1973

2. STRAUSS HW, JAMES AE, HURLEY PJ: Nuclear cerebral angiography. Usefulness in the differential diagnosis of cerebrovascular disease and tumor. *Arch Intern Med* 131: 211–216, 1973

3. WITCOFSKI RL, MAYNARD CD, ROPER TJ: Comparative analysis of accuracy of ^{99m}Tc-pertechnetate brain scan: follow-up of 1000 patients. *J Nucl Med* 8: 187–196, 1967

4. OVERTON MC, SNODGRASS SR, HAYNIE FP: Brain scans in neoplastic intracranial lesions: scanning with chlormerodrin ^{203}Hg and chlormerodrin ^{197}Hg. *JAMA* 192: 747, 1965

5. GOODRICH JK, TUTOR FT: The isotope encephalogram in brain tumor diagnosis. *J Nucl Med* 6: 541, 1965

6. WANG Y, SHEA FJ, ROSEN JA: A comparison of the accuracy of brain scanning and other procedures used for brain tumor detection. *Neurology* 15: 1117, 1965

7. CUSHING H, EISENHARDT L: *Meningiomas, Part I*. New York, Hafner Publishing Company, 1969

8. CUSHING H, EISENHARDT L: *Meningiomas, Part II.* New York, Hafner Publishing Company, 1969

9. CUSHING H: *Tumors of the Nervus Acusticus and the Syndrome of the Cerebellopontile Angle.* New York, Hafner Publishing Company, 1963

Chapter 2

Molecular Criteria for Blood-Brain Barrier Penetration

William H. Oldendorf

The term "blood-brain barrier" (BBB) implies that the brain capillary bed is impermeable. This concept originated nearly a century ago with the observation that polar dyes, following intravenous injection, stained all tissues except brain. A BBB certainly exists for this class of highly polar solutes and it prevents the distribution of these colored tracers from plasma into the extracellular fluid (ECF) of brain whereas it quickly distributes to the ECF of other tissues.

Our fund of general information, on the other hand, would allow us to infer that the BBB must be selectively permeable since certain drugs, such as barbiturates, have an immediate effect after intravenous injection, and brain metabolic substrates must also penetrate the BBB.

A great number of animal experiments (> 10,000) examining more than 150 radiolabeled substances has allowed us to characterize the molecular basis of this selective permeability of the BBB.

Capillary Characteristics

It is now generally agreed that the BBB is an effect of unique structural characteristics of brain capillaries and that the nervous system capillary is in fact the site of the BBB. These singular structural features of brain capillaries are best described in relation to general non-neural capillaries. The left portion of Fig. 2-1 shows a general capillary and the routes of exchange between blood plasma

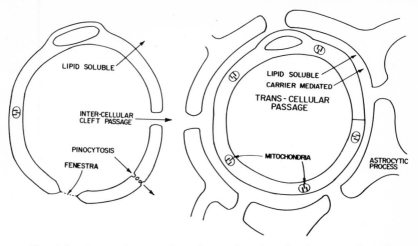

Fig. 2-1. Routes of nonspecific exchange through walls of non-neural capillaries (left) and absence of these nonspecific routes in brain capillaries (right). Brain capillaries lack open intercellular clefts, fenestrations, and pinocytotic vesicles, and contain about five times as many mitochondria, indicating apparently large metabolic work capacity. This may be related to energy-dependent unidirectional transport, such as extrusion of potassium from brain ECF.

inside the capillary with the more stationary ECF outside. Small molecules (MW <20,000–40,000) can readily diffuse along the intercellular cleft or through the tenuous membrane bridging the fenestrations. Molecules of any size (even up to several million MW) can be transported across the capillary cell by pinocytosis. This route is relatively inefficient compared to the other routes. Although solutes could exchange directly through the cell membranes and cytoplasm, the other extracellular routes are so efficient and nonspecific in their transport criteria that they mask any attempt to measure any transcellular transport that probably occurs for certain solutes.

In the brain capillary (Fig. 2-1, right) these extracellular routes of transport are, by some undetermined mechanism, closed. The intercellular clefts are sealed shut by the formation of tight junctions between adjacent cells, no fenestrations are formed, and pinocytotic vesicles are 15–20 times less numerous. Accordingly, transport across brain capillaries must take place directly through the endothelial cells of the capillary wall. BBB permeability is established by the ability of a solute to leave the plasma water, enter the inner endothelial cell membrane, leave the membrane, traverse the thin layer of cytoplasm, and repeat the penetration at the outer membrane. The chemical characteristics of a solute molecule establish the likelihood of successfully traversing the capillary cell (1).

BBB permeability can be correlated with the ability of a molecule in plasma water to detach itself from this water and enter the endothelial cell membrane. Two general characteristics seem to explain BBB permeability. One is the lipid versus water affinity of the solute. This characteristic establishes the likelihood that the plasma solute will make the transition from plasma water into membrane lipid. Thus, there is general recognition that lipid-soluble substances penetrate the BBB, and the instantaneous central effects of barbiturates and certain other centrally active drugs are explained since these drugs are, to varying degrees, appreciably soluble in lipids.

Knowing the structure of a molecule, one can estimate its water affinity. This affinity is largely determined, for un-ionized molecules, by the total hydrogen-bonding capability of the molecule. This, in turn, can be estimated by adding up the -OH and -NH$_2$ groups and less active groups (2). An ionization site on a molecule results in a large charge-dipole interaction with water and each charge site is equivalent to the hydrogen bond strength of some three to eight hydroxyl or primary amine groups.

This mechanism explains the entry of nonpolar drugs into brain but not the obvious entry of highly polar solutes, such as glucose, into brain. Glucose is so extremely water soluble that it has virtually no chance of achieving the rather great kinetic energy required to escape its bonding to water and enter the membrane lipid. Therefore, the membrane is specialized by virtue of specific protein components that have a sufficient affinity for glucose to cause it to detach from the adjacent water phase and enter the membrane. These selective proteins make certain plasma solutes, in a sense, selectively soluble in the membrane much as hemoglobin makes oxygen selectively soluble in blood plasma. These membrane proteins exhibiting specific affinities are referred to as carriers. "Carrier-mediated" BBB permeability is the second mechanism by which the barrier can be penetrated. In our work to date, we have identified seven independent BBB systems, each facilitating the BBB transport of a class of related substances.

Lipid-mediated penetration and carrier-mediated penetration can be treated separately although very similar methods are used to study both mechanisms.

Experimental Methods

We have measured in rats the BBB permeability to a large number of substances by injecting the ^{14}C-labeled substance into the carotid artery and measuring the percentage lost to brain during a single microcirculatory passage (3, 4). This is done by a rather simple technique in which a highly diffusible ^{3}H-labeled internal standard (^{3}H$_2$O) is mixed with the injected test substance. It is assumed all of the ^{3}H$_2$O remains in brain (actually only about 80% is retained) and the amount of ^{14}C versus ^3H in the brain 15 sec after injection establishes the percent uptake for the test substance.

Lipid-Mediated Brain Uptake

When the olive oil/water partition coefficient is compared to percent uptake by brain it can be established that, above a certain threshold for this coefficient (0.02–0.03), nearly complete clearance is obtained (Fig. 2-2). It is important to recognize that it is the actual oil/water partition coefficient that determines membrane penetration and not the absolute lipid solubility.

The observation that many substances having even a moderate lipid solubility relative to water are completely cleared in one pass through the brain is of considerable interest in nuclear medicine because it means that the amount of tracer delivered into a region of brain is established by the amount of blood delivered to that region, and the delivery of tracer to each small brain region, therefore, is flow limited. The initial regional distribution in brain of such a flow-limited tracer will be in proportion to regional blood flow.

We have studied the regional distribution of intravenous ^{131}I-iodoantipyrine in humans as an indicator of regional blood flow (5, 6). More recently we have studied ^{123}I-iodoantipyrine (7) because of its

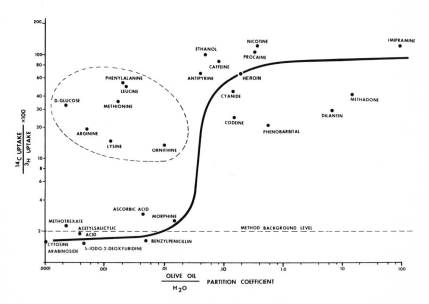

Fig. 2-2. Relation between lipid/water partition coefficient and percent uptake by brain during single microcirculatory passage. Percent uptake rises strikingly above method background (2%, horizontal dashed line) when olive oil/water partition coefficient rises above about 0.03. (Reprinted with permission from Ref. 4.)

more ideal decay characteristics for scintillation camera imaging in humans. As might be predicted, iodoantipyrine produces an image of the head in which the brain lights up more than the extracranial tissue. A large dose, together with regional counting capability, should make relative regional flow measurements possible.

Iodine-123-labeled iodoantipyrine is not ideal because ^{123}I is expensive and not widely available. A lipid-soluble (partition coefficient $>0.1-0.2$) ^{99m}Tc-labeled compound would be more desirable because of the shorter physical half-life and general availability of ^{99m}Tc in large amounts from generators. Such a tracer would probably find widespread clinical application for atraumatic display of regional blood flow in brain and in other tissues.

Nonvolatile lipid-soluble tracers have a great practical advantage over gaseous lipid-soluble tracers such as xenon because they are not lost to alveolar air after intravenous injection and thus are efficiently delivered to the periphery after cardiopulmonary passage. We have preliminary evidence (unpublished) that tracers having a very high lipid/water partition coefficient (such as ^{14}C-imipramine; partition coefficient ≈ 100) are largely sequestered in lung lipid for a considerable period of time after intravenous injection. These observations suggest that an ideal partition coefficient for intravenous bloodflow scanning would be in the range of $0.1-5.0$.

Carrier-Mediated BBB Permeability

Of greater physiological interest is carrier-mediated penetration of the BBB. The encircled group of substances on the left of Fig. 2-2 represents lipid-insoluble substances that still exhibit an appreciable clearance by brain. By adding known concentrations of unlabeled test substances to these injections we have established the saturability of these carrier-mediated uptakes whereas no such saturation effects were seen with lipid-mediated uptake. There are a finite number of carrier sites in the BBB but an essentially infinite capacity of the membrane lipid to hold lipid-soluble test substances.

At present there is only one generally available, gamma-emitting intermediary metabolite, ^{75}Se-selenomethionine, the behavior of which is virtually indistinguishable from natural methionine. We have used this tracer to demonstrate BBB saturation effects in phenylketonuric humans having very high blood phenylalanine levels (8–10). Both being neutral amino acids, phenylalanine and methionine show affinity for the same amino acid carrier site, and mutual inhibition of BBB transport is readily demonstrated.

To date, we have demonstrated the following BBB carriers (3, 11): (A) Certain hexoses—D-glucose, D-mannose, D-galactose, 2-deoxy D-glucose, and 3-O-methyl D-glucose—exhibit affinities for the same site; D-fructose and L-glucose do not. The carrier is stereospecific for D-hexoses. (B) Short-chain monocarboxylic acids—pyruvate, L-lactate and β-hydroxybutyrate, acetate, propionate, and n-butyrate—show affinities (12). (C) Of the neutral amino acids, only proline and glycine do not show measurable affinities. (D) Basic amino acids. (E) Acidic amino acids. (F) Certain purines, notably adenine. (G) Certain nucleosides, notably adenosine.

The affinity of amino acids for one of the recognizable carrier sites seems to be based on two criteria: the alpha-amino acid configuration at one end of the molecule and the net molecular charge at body pH. Each amino acid has a measurable affinity for only one carrier. Thus the net negative molecular charge of -1 of acidic amino acids seems to establish affinity for the acidic amino-acid carrier site. Similarly, the neutrals are grouped together. With the basic amino acids, their net positive charges seem to establish their common carrier affinity. This segregation, apparently on the basis of charge, suggests that it is the ionized species that is transported rather than the minor fraction of un-ionized molecules. When there is addition or removal of a proton-labile group, the carrier affinity shifts to the appropriate new carrier. Thus, amination of glutamic acid to glutamine switches its affinity from the acidic to the neutral carrier. The amino acid carriers are variably stereospecific but always prefer the L-form (11).

Uptake by the human brain of many of these substances could be studied if ^{11}C or ^{13}N were used as labels since their annihilation photon emissions could be counted externally. Despite their short half-lives, the amount of nuclide in brain after intravenous injection could easily be counted by external detectors. The physiological parameter assessed by this means would largely be BBB penetration. What happens to the labeled molecule once in brain is very difficult to assess because the only data available are the nuclide counting rates and this tells little about specific biochemical transformation except as an indicator of $^{11}CO_2$ production. Such CO_2 production could be estimated because the ^{11}C taking this pathway should be washed rapidly out of the brain. More specific assessment of the metabolic fate of a labeled compound in brain does not seem feasible by simply counting the residual radionuclide in the brain. One would have to obtain a sample of brain tissue and analyze it in some way to determine the molecular identity of the radiolabel. How this could be carried out in humans is not obvious.

Summary

The blood-brain barrier is located at the brain capillary endothelial cell and is selectively permeable. Permeability is determined by the ability of a molecule to leave the adjacent water and enter the endothelial cell membrane. This entry can be based on simple lipid solubility, in which case penetration is nonsaturable, and on specific affinities for specific carrier proteins exhibiting sufficient affinity to attract the solute away from the adjacent water. This type of membrane penetration is saturable. Seven such carrier systems have been identified. Lipid-mediated BBB penetration can be predicted quite well from the lipid/water partition coefficient, which in turn can be estimated by knowing the ionization state of the molecule and its hydrogen-bonding capability. Carrier-mediated permeability is much more difficult to predict since affinity for the various carriers is based on a number of highly specific molecular structure characteristics.

References

1. OLDENDORF WH: Blood-brain barrier permeability to drugs. *Ann Rev Pharmacol* 14: 239–248, 1974

2. STEIN WD: *The Movement of Molecules Across Cell Membranes.* New York, Academic Press, 1967

3. OLDENDORF WH: Brain uptake of radiolabeled amino acids, amines, and hexoses after arterial injection. *Am J Physiol* 221: 1629–1639, 1971

4. OLDENDORF WH: Lipid solubility and drug penetration of the blood brain barrier. *Proc Soc Exp Biol Med* 147: 813–816, 1974

5. OLDENDORF WH, KITANO M: The symmetry of I^{131} 4-iodoantipyrine uptake by brain after intravenous injection. *Neurology* 15: 994–999, 1965

6. OLDENDORF WH, KITANO M: The free passage of I^{131} antipyrine through brain as an indication of A-V shunting. *Neurology* 14: 1078–1083, 1964

7. USZLER JM, BENNETT LR, MENA I, et al: Human CNS perfusion scanning with ^{123}I iodoantypyrine. *Radiology* 115: 197–200, 1975

8. OLDENDORF WH, SISSON WB, MEHTA AC, et al: Brain uptake of selenomethionine Se-75. I. Effects of elevated blood levels of methionine and phenylalanine. *Arch Neurol* 24: 423–430, 1971

9. OLDENDORF WH, SISSON WB, SILVERSTEIN A: Brain uptake of selenomethionine Se-75. II. Reduced brain uptake of selenomethionine Se-75 in phenylketonuria. *Arch Neurol* 24: 524–528, 1971

10. OLDENDORF WH: Saturation of blood brain barrier transport of amino acids in phenylketonuria. *Arch Neurol* 28: 45-48, 1973

11. OLDENDORF WH: Stereospecificity of blood-brain permeability to amino acids. *Am J Physiol* 224: 967–969, 1973

12. OLDENDORF WH: Carrier-mediated blood-brain barrier transport of short-chain monocarboxylic organic acids. *Am J Physiol* 224: 1450–1453, 1973

Chapter 3

New Short-Lived Radiopharmaceuticals for CNS Studies

Michael J. Welch, John O. Eichling,
Maria G. Straatmann, Marcus E. Raichle,
and Michel M. Ter-Pogossian

The radiopharmaceuticals currently used in neuronuclear medicine have been designed as compounds that demonstrate the breakdown of the blood-brain barrier (*1*), assess cerebrospinal fluid pathways (*2*), or assess regional cerebral blood flow (*3*). The first of these applications utilizes radiopharmaceuticals that do not penetrate the intact blood-brain barrier, the second utilizes either labeled proteins or chelates, while the third most commonly utilizes intra-arterial injections of dissolved ^{133}Xe.

With the introduction of the small medical cyclotron (*4, 5*), radionuclides have become available that allow the synthesis and use of radiopharmaceuticals that are in fact metabolites. In this chapter we will discuss the use of radiopharmaceuticals labeled with the short-lived positron-emitting nuclides ^{15}O (half-life, 2.04 min), ^{13}N (half-life, 9.96 min), and ^{11}C (half-life, 20.3 min) in CNS studies. The further potential of compounds labeled with these nuclides as well as ^{18}F (half-life, 1.89 hr) used in conjunction with newer tomographic imaging techniques (Chapter 7) will be discussed, as will the advantages of other cyclotron-produced inert gases compared to those of ^{133}Xe.

We have used ^{15}O-labeled water, oxyhemoglobin, and car-boxyhemoglobin for the measurement of regional blood flow, oxygen metabolism, and blood volume. These compounds are all prepared from $O^{15}O$ obtained by deuteron irradiation of nitrogen containing a trace of oxygen. The chemistry of the recoiling oxygen atom formed by the $^{14}N(d,n)^{15}O$ nuclear reaction is such that its reactivity with oxygen and carbon dioxide is several orders of magnitude greater than its reactivity with nitrogen (6). This allows the formation of $O^{15}O$ of very high specific activity in nitrogen carrier gas. The labeled oxygen is converted into carbon dioxide by passage through a furnace containing activated charcoal maintained at 400°C, and into carbon monoxide by passage through a similar furnace maintained at 1,125°C. The ^{15}O-labeled gases are then bubbled through blood as shown in Fig. 3-1. Oxygen and carbon monoxide are purified from any traces of

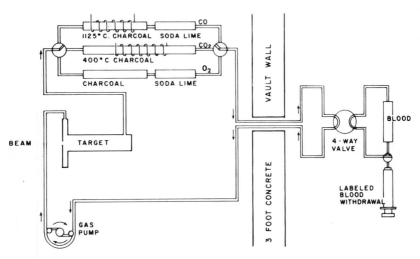

Fig. 3-1. Schematic diagram of system used to produce ^{15}O-oxyhemoglobin, ^{15}O-carboxyhemoglobin, and $H_2{}^{15}O$.

^{15}O-carbon dioxide by passage through a soda lime trap and, when dissolved in blood, form oxyhemoglobin and carboxyhemoglobin, respectively. Labeled carbon dioxide dissolves in the blood and is rapidly converted to labeled water through the reaction sequence:

$$CO^{15}O + H_2O \rightleftarrows H_2CO_2{}^{15}O \rightleftarrows CO_2 + H_2{}^{15}O.$$

Each time carbonic acid forms and dissociates, there is about a 0.33 probability that the oxygen will be on the water molecule. In blood this reaction is very fast because of the presence of the enzyme carbonic anhydrase, and no CO^{15}O can be detected at equilibrium, which is reached in less than 2 min (7, 8).

Using the system shown in Fig. 3-1 with solenoid valves to alter the direction of flow of the gas, solutions of ^{15}O-labeled carboxyhemoglobin and oxyhemoglobin containing approximately 1 mCi/cc can be prepared in about 5 min, and tens of mCi/cc of ^{15}O-labeled water in about 2 min.

These radiopharmaceuticals are currently being used to measure regional cerebral blood flow, regional cerebral oxygen metabolism, and regional cerebral blood volume. Intra-arterial injections are used and measurements are made with the multiprobe system shown in Fig. 3-2. The 26-probe system has 13 collimated NaI(Tl) detectors positioned over each hemisphere of the brain and the parameters listed above are calculated for each of the 13 regions. Typical curves for the transit of the three ^{15}O-labeled tracers are shown in Fig. 3-3.

Regional cerebral blood flow (rCBF). Regional cerebral blood flow is determined by analysis of the washout curve for labeled water (9). In the original work a 10-min washout was used. However, an index of flow enabling blood flow to be assessed by utilizing only the first 90 sec of the washout curve has since been developed (10). Specifically, the index, I_F, is given by the equation:

$$I_F = 100 \ln(A_{15}/A_{75}) \tag{1}$$

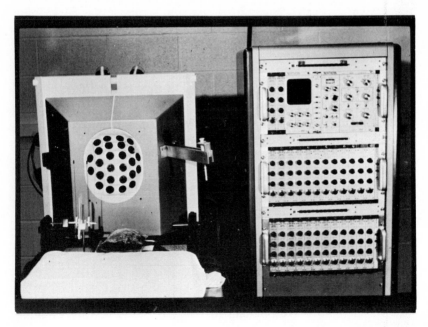

Fig. 3-2. Multiprobe system for studying ^{15}O-labeled tracers in brain.

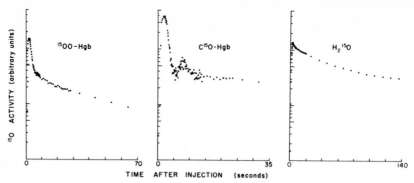

Fig. 3-3. Typical curves obtained over head following intracarotid injection of three ^{15}O-labeled tracers.

where A_{15} and A_{75} are counting rates observed at 15 and 75 sec after injection. Data from 75 studies on humans yielded the regression:

$$rCBF \text{ (ml/100 gm tissue/min)} = 0.71 \, I_F + 4.4 \quad (r = -0.98). \quad (2)$$

By using this index, rCBF measurements can be carried out very rapidly with a significant reduction of catheter dwell time.

Oxygen metabolism. Oxygen-15-labeled oxyhemoglobin is used for studies of oxygen metabolism. Following intra-arterial injection a certain fraction, b, of ^{15}O-oxyhemoglobin is extracted by brain from the blood. We estimate the fraction, b, by extrapolating the slow phase of the washout curve back to the point of intersection with a line drawn vertically down from the maximum of the curve, and comparing the point of intersection to the maximum height of the curve (see Fig. 3-6). The ratio of these two heights is b. The regional cerebral oxygen metabolism rate, rCMO$_2$, is then calculated from:

$$rCMO_2 \text{ (mmole/100 gm/min)} = b \times rCBF \times [O_2] \quad (3)$$

where $[O_2]$ is oxygen concentration measured in a carotid blood sample (mmole/ml) (*11*). Recent studies in our laboratory on rhesus monkeys have shown good agreement between oxygen utilization measured by this technique and by conventional arterial-venous-difference methods (*12*).

Regional cerebral blood volume. Regional cerebral blood volume is calculated by comparing the mean transit times for water and carboxyhemoglobin, $\bar{t}_{H_2O}$ and $\bar{t}_{RBC}$, using the relationships:

$$F/W_{H_2O} = F/\rho V_{H_2O} = \lambda'_{H_2O}/\rho \bar{t}_{H_2O} = \lambda_{H_2O}/\bar{t}_{H_2O} \quad (4)$$
$$F/V_{RBC} = 1/\bar{t}_{RBC}. \quad (5)$$

Here F is the blood flow (ml/min); V_{H_2O} and V_{RBC} are distribution volumes (ml) for water and red blood cells; W_{H_2O} is the weight of brain tissue (gm) corresponding to V_{H_2O}; ρ is the density of brain tissue; λ'_{H_2O} is the dimensionless partition coefficient; and $\lambda_{H_2O} =$

0.95 ml/gm (13) is the partition coefficient for water between brain tissue and blood. The method of measuring t is based on the central volume principle, according to which

$$\bar{t} = (1/H_0) \int_0^\infty C \, dt \tag{6}$$

where H_0 is the maximum counting rate observed and $\int_0^\infty C \, dt$ is the area under the first-pass portion of the curve. The curve was extrapolated assuming a functional form $C = At^{-m}$, where A and m are adjustable parameters chosen to give a best fit to the data (see Fig. 3-8). If f = cerebral hematocrit/large vessel hematocrit, regional cerebral blood volume, V_{RBC} or rCBV, is given by:

$$rCBV \text{ (ml/100 gm)} = (\lambda_{H_2O} \times \bar{t}_{RBC})/(\bar{t}_{H_2O} \times f). \tag{7}$$

A value for f can be obtained by techniques employing ^{11}C-labeled methyl albumin discussed below, and therefore rCBV can be calculated.

Studies have been carried out to measure these three physiological parameters with ^{15}O-labeled radiopharmaceuticals on several groups of patients (14–16).

Nitrogen-13

Solutions containing labeled nitrogen gas have been prepared and show promise in rCBF measurement because of the lower lipid solubility of N_2 when compared to xenon (17). This is perhaps an important characteristic for a tracer used to measure cerebral blood flow, since it has been shown that the lipid content of cerebral tissue varies greatly with pathology (18). The radionuclide used in the preparation of the $N^{13}N$ has generally been prepared by the $^{12}C(d,n)^{13}N$ nuclear reaction. At Hammersmith Hospital (19) carbon granules supported by a graphite grid are used as the target material. After producing ^{13}N in a hydrogen carrier gas, the gas is passed over cupric oxide to convert the hydrogen to water. The nitrogen is then dissolved in saline prior to injection. Because of the limited solubility of nitrogen, it is difficult to produce solutions of high activity by this method.

If nitrogen atoms are formed in gaseous carbon monoxide or carbon dioxide, these atoms do not react with the target molecules, but instead react with traces of molecular nitrogen always present in these gases as impurities (20). The overall reaction scheme is:

$$^{13}N + N_2 \rightarrow N^{13}N^* + N$$
$$N^{13}N^* + CO_2 \text{ (or } O_2 \text{ or CO)} \rightarrow N^{13}N$$
$$N^{13}N^* + CO_2 \text{ (or } O_2 + CO)} \rightarrow N^{13}NO$$

with an excited form of molecular nitrogen ($N^{13}N^*$) being formed as an intermediate. Under normal irradiation conditions the nitrous oxide is radiolytically decomposed to nitrogen by the cyclotron beam. Solutions of $N^{13}N$ are prepared after passing the gas over cupric oxide to convert carbon monoxide (which is also formed radiolytically from carbon dioxide), into carbon dioxide and then absorbing the CO_2 in a soda lime trap prior to dissolution of the nitrogen in saline.

We have also used ^{13}N-labeled ammonia for CNS studies. This compound is produced for medical use by bombarding aluminum carbide with deuterons $[^{12}C(d,n)^{13}N]$ (21, 22). The aluminum carbide is then dissolved in acid producing dissolved ^{13}N-ammonia in solution. The solution is made basic to evolve the ammonia as a gas, which is then distilled and redissolved in a small volume of acid. One disadvantage of this technique is that the chemist may receive a rather large radiation dose from activated aluminum products (^{28}Al) during the procedure. An alternative production method utilizes deuteron bombardment of a gaseous methane target (23, 24). These two methods suffer the common disadvantage that significant amounts of carrier ammonia may be produced because of nitrogen contamination of the target. Perhaps the best method of ammonia production involves the bombardment of water with protons to form ^{13}N by the $^{16}O(p,\alpha)^{13}N$ nuclear reaction, followed by the reduction of the ^{13}N compounds to ammonia with titanous chloride (25). This method produces a high purity radiopharmaceutical very rapidly. However, the Washington University Medical School cyclotron does not produce a proton beam to permit use of this method.

We have studied the effects of blood pH on brain, blood, and liver concentrations of injected ^{13}N-ammonia in dogs (21). The tracer was injected intravenously, and brain and liver activities were monitored with external probes while blood concentration was monitored by sample counting techniques. Prior to injection, blood pH was altered by infusion of 0.2 M sodium hydroxide or acetic acid. It was found that the liver/blood, brain/blood, and brain/liver ratios all increased at elevated pH (~7.6), while the reverse was true at lowered pH (~6.9). The largest changes were observed in the blood/brain ratio. It should be noted that the brain activity levels were constant after 2 min. This should permit accurate determination of brain-ammonia levels with tomographic techniques discussed later in this chapter.

Inert Gases

In addition to ^{13}N, several other radioactive gases that may be useful for rCBF studies can be prepared with a medical cyclotron. These include a number of inert gases having more favorable decay characteristics than ^{133}Xe. A list of these gases and a summary of their properties is given in Table 3-1.

TABLE 3-1. Short-Lived Inert Gas Radionuclides

Isotope	Half-life	Major radiations (MeV)	Possible means of production
^{123}Xe	2.08 hr	0.149 0.511 (β^+)	^{122}Te$(\alpha,3n)^{123}$Xe ^{123}Te$(^3$He,3n$)^{123}$Xe ^{127}I$(p,5n)^{123}$Xe
^{135}Xe	9.21 hr	0.250	^{134}Xe$(n,\gamma)^{135}$Xe
^{77}Kr	1.2 hr	0.511 (β^+)	^{76}Se$(\alpha,3n)^{77}$Kr
^{81m}Kr	13 sec	0.190	Daughter of ^{81}Rb* (half-life = 4.9 hr)
^{85m}Kr	4.4 hr	0.150	^{82}Se$(\alpha,n)^{85m}$Kr

* Produced by the ^{81}Br$(\alpha,4n)$ or ^{81}Br$(^3$He,3n$)$ reactions.

Carbon-11

Several ^{11}C-labeled compounds have been used to assess various cerebral parameters. Carbon-11-labeled bicarbonate to study regional pH (26), ^{11}C-glucose and ^{11}C-acetoacetate to study metabolism (27, 28), various alcohols to study blood-brain barrier permeability (29), and ^{11}C-proteins to study brain hematocrit (30) will be discussed.

Carbon-11 is produced in high yields by bombarding boron with deuterons of energy greater than 6 MeV. Boric oxide is melted into a molybdenum mesh and mounted perpendicular to the cyclotron beam. The energy of deposition of the beam melts the boric oxide, releasing ^{11}C produced by the ^{10}B$(d,n)^{11}$C reaction as carbon monoxide, which is swept out of the target chamber using helium carrier gas (6, 31). The activity is built up in a closed circulating system similar to that used for ^{15}O production. If ^{11}C-carbon dioxide is required, a small percent of oxygen is added to the circulating gas and the carbon monoxide is radiolytically oxidized to carbon dioxide.

$$O_2 \xrightarrow{\text{radiation}} 2O$$
$$^{11}CO + O \rightarrow {}^{11}CO_2$$

Injectable bicarbonate solutions are prepared by bubbling the gas through an aliquot of the subject's blood.

Intracellular pH (pHi). In the past the only satisfactory method for determining intracellular pH in the brain was to measure HCO_3^- concentration in the brain tissue of small animals sacrificed before measurement (32). We have developed techniques employing ^{11}C-labeled bicarbonate and external detectors for in vivo measurements of this parameter (26).

The method utilizes external residue detection and requires the serial measurement of the mean transit time of blood containing the two tracers, ^{15}O-labeled water and ^{11}C-labeled carbon dioxide. Under the condition of constant cerebral blood flow, the total CO_2 content per gram of brain tissue, TCO_2, can be obtained from the relationship:

$$TCO_2\text{(mmole/kg)} = \lambda_{H_2O} \times \bar{t}_{CO_2} \times BCO_2/\bar{t}_{H_2O} \qquad (8)$$

where λ_{H_2O} is the mean tissue-blood equilibrium partition coefficient of water (0.95 ml/gm), $\bar{t}_{CO_2}$ and $\bar{t}_{H_2O}$ are the mean transit times of the two tracers, and BCO_2 (mmole/liter) is the total CO_2 content of the blood, including carbamino CO_2, bicarbonate ion, and dissolved CO_2. The intracellular HCO_3^- concentration, in meq/liter can then be computed from the equations:

$$[HCO_3^-]_t = TCO_2 - (P_tCO_2 \times S_1) \qquad (9)$$
$$[HCO_3^-]_i = ([HCO_3^-]_t - V_{ecf}[HCO_3^-]_{csf})/V_i \qquad (10)$$

where $[HCO_3^-]_t$, $[HCO_3^-]_i$, and $[HCO_3^-]_{csf}$ denote the brain tissue bicarbonate concentration (meq/kg of tissue), the intracellular bicarbonate concentration (meq/kg of intracellular water), and the cerebrospinal fluid (CSF) bicarbonate concentration (meq/kg of CSF), respectively. The mean tissue CO_2 tension, P_tCO_2, was obtained from the measured arteriovenous P_aCO_2 differences. The solubility coefficient for CO_2 in whole brain tissue (S_1) was assumed to be 0.0292 (mmoles/kg tissue/mm Hg) (32). On the basis of measurements by others (32, 33), we assumed the extracellular fluid volume (V_{ecf}) to be 15% and the intracellular water volume (V_i) to be 64% of total tissue mass.

From this the pHi can be calculated using the Henderson-Hasselbach equation:

$$pHi = 6.12 + \{log[HCO_3^-]_i/(P_tCO_2 \times S_2)\} \qquad (11)$$

where S_2 is the solubility coefficient of CO_2 in intracellular water and equal to 0.0314 mmoles/kg intracellular water/mm Hg (32).

This method gives values of pHi in the range of 7.24–7.05 for an arterial CO_2 tension range of 30–55 mm Hg with a mean pHi of 7.13 for an arterial CO_2 tension of 40 mm Hg. These preliminary data are in good agreement with previously reported values using radically different means to measure $[HCO_3^-]_i$ (34).

Brain metabolism. We have employed ^{11}C-labeled glucose (35, 36) to assess regional brain metabolism of glucose. Carbon-11-labeled glucose is prepared by photosynthesis using Swiss chard leaves. After production of ^{11}C-carbon dioxide from a boric oxide target as described previously, the carbon dioxide in the carrier gas is passed over a light-starved Swiss chard leaf contained in a glass vessel and illuminated using a Microlite daylight white lamp. After 20 min of photosynthesis, which is carried out while the activity is still being produced, the leaf is removed from the chamber and the sugars extracted. Glucose, fructose, sucrose, and sugar phosphates are extracted with ethanol, then the sucrose and phosphates are hydrolyzed with acid, and finally the solution is boiled and filtered prior to purification. Chromatography using Woelm magnesium silicate (activity grade 1) enriches the glucose-fructose mixture from about 65% glucose to about 85% glucose in approximately 25 min. The presence of small amounts of fructose does not affect CNS studies because fructose does not cross the blood-brain barrier (Chapter 2).

A complete glucose/fructose separation can be obtained with a high-performance carbohydrate column (μ-Bondapak, Waters Associates, Inc., Milford, Mass.). The separation can be accomplished in less than 30 min for sample volumes as large as 2 cc. A problem with this technique is that the eluting solvent contains 65% acetonitrile, which must be removed before injection. We therefore use (and recommend) the technique only for quality control purposes.

Carbon-11-labeled glucose prepared in this manner has been used for in vivo measurement of brain-glucose transport kinetics and metabolism in the rhesus monkey and in a limited number of patients. The labeled compound was injected intravenously as a bolus. Radioactivity in the head and in arterial blood was monitored continuously, the latter utilizing an indwelling peripheral arterial catheter for a data collection period of 2–3 min. A second intravenous injection of ^{15}O-carboxyhemoglobin was used to obtain a correction for radioactivity in blood in the head. The method was tested in nine phencyclidine-anesthetized monkeys whose cerebral glucose metabolism (CMRGlu) was also measured by standard methods employing the Fick principle. A highly significant correlation ($r = 0.929$) was found between the tracer and standard methods of measuring CMRGlu (27).

One problem in the measurement of glucose metabolism with ^{11}C-glucose is the egress of [11]CO_2 produced by glucose metabolism. A more suitable compound would therefore be an analog that is transported as glucose but then trapped intracellularly as an intermediate in the glycolytic cycle. Three potentially useful compounds with this property are 2-deoxy-D-glucose (37), 2-deoxy-2-fluoro-D-glucose (38), and 3-deoxy-3-fluoro-glucose (39). It should be possible to produce 2-deoxy-2-fluoro-glucose with ^{18}F using $CF_3O^{18}F$ as the fluorinating agent (40). Treatment of 3,4,6-tri-O-acetal-D-glucal with CF_3OF in freon-11 solvent at $-70°C$ gives a mixture of 2-deoxy-2-fluoro derivatives that, on acid hydrolysis, yields 2-deoxy-2-fluoro-glucose as shown in Fig. 3-4.

In order to study brain metabolism of a ketogenic substrate in subjects with abnormal brain metabolism, we have also synthesized ^{11}C-labeled acetoacetic acid. This synthesis utilizes a method of prep-

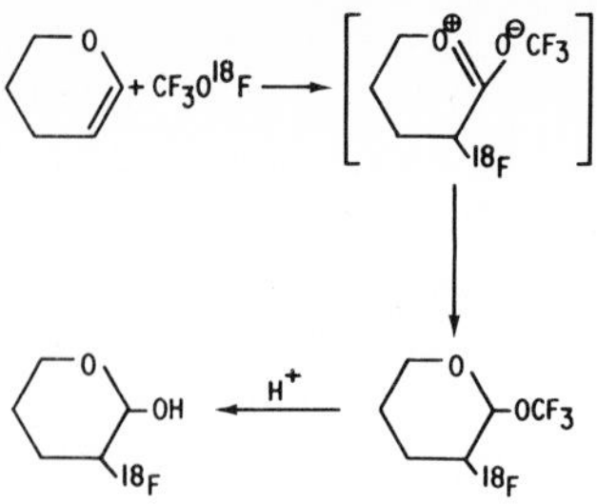

Fig. 3-4. Reaction sequence for production of ^{18}F-labeled glucose analog, 2-deoxy-2-fluoro-glucose.

aration of solutions of enolate anions developed by House and coworkers specifically for use with ^{11}C (*41, 42*). In this preparation a lithium enolate anion is generated by the reaction of the enol acetate of a ketone with methyl lithium in a nonporotic solvent. The anion generated from isopropenyl acetate in this manner is used to trap ^{11}C-labeled carbon dioxide resulting in the formation of the desired ^{11}C-labeled acetoacetate.

In the actual preparation, the enolate anion can be produced in advance of the radioactive ^{11}CO$_2$ because of its stability. This preparation is carried out by adding isopropenyl acetate to methyl lithium in dry ether and stirring for approximately 45 min. After production of ^{11}CO$_2$ the enolate anion and the labeled carbon dioxide are shaken for 20 min, and after acidification the acetoacetic acid is purified and separated using a small column of Amberlite CG-4B ion exchange resin eluted with distilled water. The total synthesis takes 40 min with an overall chemical yield of approximately 50%.

Blood-brain barrier permeability studies. Radiolabeled water is assumed to equilibrate with the brain tissue during a single capillary transit. Water has therefore been used as a standard for the evaluation of blood-brain barrier (BBB) permeability (Chapter 2). However, recent investigations have shown that water does not freely equilibrate with the exchangeable water of the brain (*43, 44*). Labeled ethanol has been proposed as a freely diffusible tracer (*45*) and we have therefore synthesized a series of labeled alcohols to investigate their extraction during a single capillary transit in the rhesus monkey.

Carbon-11-labeled methanol was synthesized by the reduction of ^{11}CO$_2$ prepared as described above. Radiochemical purity analysis for this and all the other alcohols was carried out by radio-gas-partition chromatography using a 6-mm o.d. aluminum column packed with Poropak-Q (Waters Associates Inc., Milford, Mass.) and operated between 80° and 200°C at a carrier helium flow rate of approximately 1 cc/min. Counting measurements were done with an internal flow proportional counter and data were analyzed by a small laboratory computer (LINC) that had been programmed to integrate peaks and to correct for radioactive decay, background, and flow rate variations.

N-butanol was prepared by carboxylation of the appropriate Grignard reagent followed by reduction with lithium aluminum hydride.

$$CH_3(CH_2)_2MgCl + {}^{11}CO_2 \rightarrow CH_3(CH_2)_2{}^{11}C \overset{\displaystyle O}{\underset{\displaystyle MgCl}{\diagup\diagdown}}$$

$$CH_3(CH_2)_2{}^{11}C \overset{\displaystyle O}{\underset{\displaystyle MgCl}{\diagup\diagdown}} \xrightarrow{\text{LiAlH}_4} CH_3(CH_2)_2{}^{11}CH_2OH$$

The reaction was carried out in ether and the reaction mixture was acidified and, after separation of the aqueous layer, neutralized. The insoluble hydroxides were removed by filtration. A typical chromatogram for n-butanol is shown in Fig. 3-5. The only impurity is a trace of ^{11}C-methanol formed by the reduction of unreacted carbon dioxide.

We also attempted to produce ethanol by a similar reaction scheme.

$$CH_3X + {}^{11}CO_2 \rightarrow CH_3{}^{11}C \overset{\displaystyle X}{\underset{\displaystyle O}{\diagup\diagdown}} \xrightarrow{\text{LiAlH}_4} CH_3{}^{11}CH_2OH$$

where X = MgCl, MgBr, MgI, or Li. It was found that large amounts of isopropanol were formed with methyl magnesium chloride and methyl lithium, presumably by the reaction:

$$2CH_3X + {}^{11}CO_2 \rightarrow (CH_3)_2{}^{11}C \overset{\displaystyle OX}{\underset{\displaystyle OX}{\diagup\diagdown}} \xrightarrow{\text{LiAlH}_4} (CH_3)_2{}^{11}CHOH.$$

Only by using methyl magnesium bromide could high specific activity ethanol be prepared. With methyl lithium, isopropanol was formed in such high yields that this method was used to produce isopropanol. Using the iodide, a mixture of methanol, ethanol, and isopropanol was always formed, but the reaction sequence was too slow to allow this to be used for ethanol production.

Injections of ^{11}C-labeled alcohol (0.2-ml solution) were made into the internal carotid artery of adult rhesus monkeys and the time

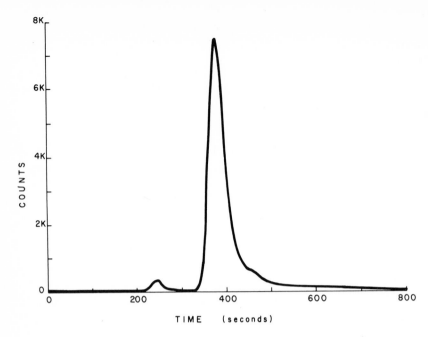

TIME (seconds)

Fig. 3-5. Typical chromatogram of ^{11}C-butanol. Small amount of impurity is $^{11}CH_3OH$.

course of the tracer monitored by means of a collimated 3-in.-diam × 2-in.-thick NaI(Tl) detector positioned over the animal's head. In each study samples of $H_2{}^{15}O$ and the labeled alcohol were injected consecutively with the water being used to determine blood flow. Typical curves are shown in Fig. 3-6. Extraction fractions at normal (50 ml/100 gm/min) and high (100 ml/100 gm/min) brain blood flows are given in Table 3-2. Labeled n-butanol appeared to be completely extracted at flow rates of 50–100 ml/100 gm/min. For the other tracers we assumed the following relationship, derived by Crone, between blood flow, F, and the extraction fraction, E (46).

TABLE 3-2. Extraction Percentages for Brain of Various (OH)-Containing Substrates

Flow (ml/min/100 gm)	Compound				
	Water %	Methanol %	Ethanol %	Isopropanol %	n-Butanol %
50	93.5	92.8	97.6	99.8	~100
100	74.4	70.5	85.3	93.2	~100

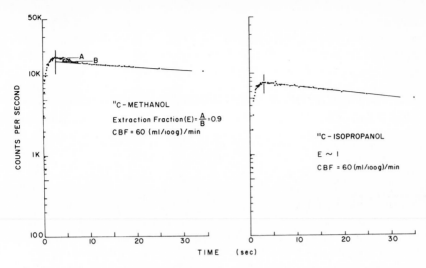

Fig. 3-6. Curves obtained after injection of ^{11}C-methanol and ^{11}C-isopropanol into internal carotid artery of rhesus monkey.

$$\ln(1 - E) = - (PS/F) + K. \qquad (12)$$

Here P is the capillary permeability (ml/min/cm²), S is the capillary surface area (cm²), and K is a constant. For the various agents tested we obtained the following results:

Water: $\ln(1 - E) = -(136/F) - 0.002$ (r = 0.98) (13)
Methanol: $\ln(1 - E) = -(141/F) - 0.19$ (r = 0.96) (14)
Ethanol: $\ln(1 - E) = -(181/F) - 0.11$ (r = 0.96) (15)
Isopropanol: $\ln(1 - E) = -(370/F) + 1.01$ (r = 0.96). (16)

Assuming a constant surface area, S, the relative capillary permeabilities for water, methanol, ethanol, and isopropanol were calculated to be 1, 1.06, 1.39, and 2.8, respectively. For n-butanol, P must be much larger, but the relative value could not be estimated since $E \approx 1$ for all measurements. The increasing order of the permeabilities noted above parallels the increase in lipid solubilities (measured by the oil/water partition coefficient) for these compounds (47; Chapter 2). Our data suggest that ethanol may be preferable to water as a standard in studies of BBB permeability because of its greater permeability, but a higher alcohol may be even better.

Cerebral hematocrit. We have used ^{11}C-labeled methyl albumin to measure cerebral hematocrit (48). The ^{11}C-labeled albumin was prepared by an adaptation of the method described by Rice and Means for the production of ^{14}C-labeled proteins (49). In this procedure ^{11}C-labeled methanol, produced as previously described, is first catalytically oxidized to formaldehyde by an adaptation of a procedure developed by Christman, et al (50). The ¹¹C-methanol is passed through a furnace maintained at 375°C containing an iron/molybdenum catalyst with a slow flow of oxygen as a transport gas. The formaldehyde is then trapped at ice temperature and evaporated to a minimum volume (0.2 cc) in borate buffer at pH 8. This solution is added to between 2 and 10 mg of albumin in 0.3 ml of borate buffer. After 2 min, 10 ml of 0.1 M sodium borohydride is added and the albumin is methylated according to the reaction sequence:

$$\text{R—NH}_2 + \text{H}_2{}^{11}\text{CO} \xrightarrow[\text{NaBH}_4]{} \text{R—}\overset{\text{H}}{\text{N}}\text{—}{}^{11}\text{CH}_3.$$

The albumin is purified by high-pressure liquid chromatography using a 60-cm-long × 1-cm-diam stainless steel column filled with Hydrogel-IV (Waters Associates, Milford, Mass.), eluted with deionized distilled water at a flow rate of 2.5 ml/min. The labeled protein separates completely from other ¹¹C-compounds very rapidly. A typical chromatogram of a preparation is shown in Fig. 3-7. The solution

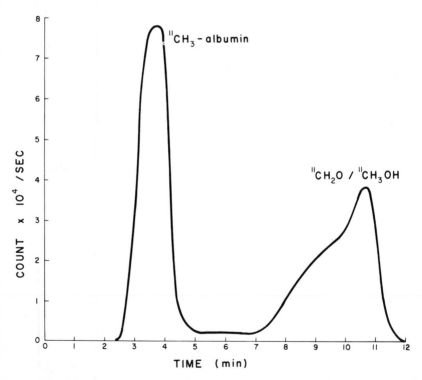

Fig. 3-7. Separation used to purify ¹¹CH₃-albumin from unreacted ¹¹CH₂O and ¹¹CH₃OH.

containing ^{11}C-protein is then passed through a Millipore filter and made isotonic for injection.

We have performed studies on rhesus monkeys employing ^{11}C-labeled albumin to measure cerebral hematocrit. We first injected ^{15}O-carboxyhemoglobin to measure RBC flow as described earlier. Then a 0.2-ml solution of labeled albumin was injected into the carotid artery. Typical curves for the two tracers are shown in Fig. 3-8, along with an illustration of the method used to calculate mean transit times, $\bar{t}$ (Eq. 6).

The calculation of cerebral hematocrit, Hct_c, was as follows. For the ^{15}O-carboxyhemoglobin data:

$$\bar{t}_{RBC} = V_{RBC}/F_{RBC} = (Hct_c \times V_c)/(Hct_{LV} \times F) \qquad (17)$$

where V_{RBC} is the red cell distribution volume, F_{RBC} is the red cell flow to the brain, V_c is the brain blood volume, F is the brain blood flow, and Hct_{LV} is the large vessel hematocrit. Applying the same principle to the transport of labeled plasma:

$$\bar{t}_p = (1 - Hct_c)V_c/\{(1 - Hct_{LV})F\}. \qquad (18)$$

Assuming constant flow, F,

$$Hct_c/Hct_{LV} = 1/\{(\bar{t}_p/\bar{t}_{RBC})(1 - Hct_{LV}) + Hct_{LV}\} \qquad (19)$$

which enables us to calculate the ratio of cerebral to large vessel hematocrit.

We measured the hematocrit ratio at normal and increased cerebral blood flows, the latter produced by inhalation of 10% CO_2. CBF was measured for each determination using $H_2{}^{15}O$ as described earlier. We found the ratio to increase with blood flow as:

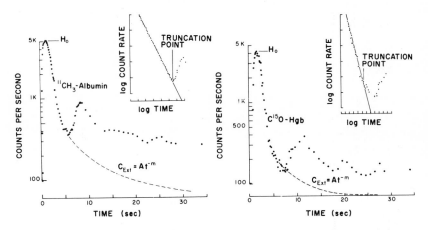

Fig. 3-8. Curves obtained following intracarotid injection of ^{11}CH$_3$-albumin and C^{15}O hemoglobin in carotid artery of rhesus monkey. Method of extrapolating curves after recirculation time is shown in inset.

$$(Hct_c/Hct_{LV}) = 0.0015 \, CBF + 0.84 \qquad (r = 0.76). \qquad (20)$$

At normal flow (CBF = 50 ml/100 gm/min) the average ratio was 0.92. The variation with flow can be explained if, in small vessels, red cells exhibit axial streaming and tend to move toward the center of the vessel. At higher flows the vessel diameter increases and thus there is less axial streaming.

Quality Control of Short-Lived Radiopharmaceuticals

Radiochemical purity is essential in most of the studies we have discussed. For example, a small amount of $H_2{}^{15}O$ impurity in ^{15}O-oxyhemoglobin will increase the extraction fraction and therefore the calculated oxygen utilization, and $H_2{}^{15}O$ impurities in ^{15}O-carboxyhemoglobin increase the measured transit time and therefore the calculated red cell volume. As discussed in the section on alcohols, even one of the simplest of chemical reactions can lead to mixed products when carrier-free materials are used. Purity checks are therefore carried out on all the products.

In the case of ^{15}O-oxyhemoglobin or ^{15}O-carboxyhemoglobin an aliquot of blood is centrifuged to separate the plasma and red cells. These are counted to check for the presence of $H_2{}^{15}O$, which will appear in the plasma. For all other radiopharmaceuticals either gas or liquid chromatographic techniques were used to measure the purity of each sample. With short-lived radiopharmaceuticals, fast separation techniques must be employed both for preparation and purity checks of the product. The two chromatographic systems used in our laboratory are shown schematically in Fig. 3-9.

Tomography and Equilibrium Imaging

Several of the measurements described here require intra-arterial injections to minimize interference from concentrations of activity in tissues overlying the brain. However, as discussed in Chapters 4 and 7, new tomographic imaging techniques make it possible to accurately quantitate activity inside the head in the presence of such overlying activity. A restriction on the use of tomographic techniques at present is that a single image requires several minutes of data collection, so that dynamic analysis is not possible. However, useful measurements may still be possible from observations of static equilibrium distributions. For example, regional blood volume and cerebral hematocrit could be determined from combined measurements of the equilibrium concentration of a circulating tracer in the brain and the concentration of activity in peripheral blood samples.

Such measurements require continuous infusion or inhalation

techniques, similar to those that have been employed for CNS studies with ^{133}Xe *(51, 52)*. Continuous inhalation of C^{15}O, CO^{15}O, and O^{15}O with tomographic imaging techniques has been suggested by Jones, et al *(53;* see also Fig. 4-4) for observation of major vessel distribution, vascularity and extravascular water turnover, and oxygen utilization, respectively. It should also be noted that a comparison of equilibrium distributions of H$_2$^{15}O and a highly lipid-soluble material such as ^{11}C-butanol should provide a method for assessing brain lipid content.

The methods described earlier for determining pHi were based on transit time determinations. It may also be possible to estimate pHi from equilibrium distributions of H^{11}CO$_3$$^-$. It has also been shown that a series of amines equilibrate in the lung at concentrations that are very dependent on pHi *(54)*. Amines having pH-sensitive tissue/blood ratios include nicotine, pentylamine, quinine, and benzylamine, and measurement of equilibrium concentrations of these substances should be useful for estimating pHi. It should be possible to label nicotine with ^{11}C by the method described earlier for

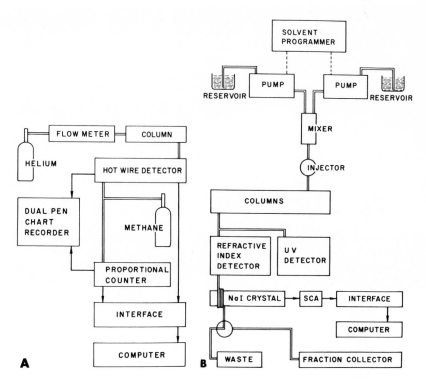

Fig. 3-9. Radiochromatographic systems used for quality control of short-lived radiopharmaceuticals. (A) Gas chromatographic system; (B) liquid chromatographic system.

methylating proteins. Pentylamine and benzylamine could be labeled with ^{13}N by reacting carrier-free ^{13}N-ammonia with the corresponding chloride.

An interesting study in which the uptake of various psychotropic drugs in the brain was measured using ^{11}C-diazepam, ^{11}C-imipramine, and ^{11}C-chlorpromazine prepared by formaldehyde/formic acid methylation has recently been described (55). Differences were observed in the uptake between psychotic patients and normals. Carbon-11-labeled psychotropic drugs may also have some applications when used in conjunction with modern tomographic techniques.

Acknowledgment

This work was supported by USPHS Grant 5-P01-HL13851.

References

1. HOLMAN B: The blood brain barrier. Anatomy and physiology. In *Progress in Nuclear Medicine,* vol 1, Potchen EJ, McCready VR, eds, Baltimore, University Park Press, 1972, pp 236–247

2. HOLMAN BL, Davis DO: Radioisotope assessment of cerebrospinal fluid pathways. In *Progress in Nuclear Medicine,* vol 1, Potchen EJ, McCready VR, eds, Baltimore, University Park Press, 1972, pp 359–375

3. LASSEN NA, INGVAR DH: Radioisotopic assessment of regional cerebral blood flow. In *Progress in Nuclear Medicine,* vol 1, Potchen EJ, McCready VR, eds, Baltimore, University Park Press, 1972, pp 376–409

4. TER-POGOSSIAN MM, WAGNER HN: A new look at the cyclotron for making short-lived isotopes. *Nucleonics* 24:40–57, 1966

5. GLASS HI, SILVESTER DJ: Cyclotrons in nuclear medicine. *Br J Radiol* 43: 489–601, 1970

6. WELCH MJ, TER-POGOSSIAN MM: Preparation of short half-lived radioactive gases for medical studies. *Radiat Res* 36: 580–587, 1968

7. WELCH MJ, LIFTON JF, TER-POGOSSIAN MM: Preparation of millicurie quantities of ^{15}O-labeled water. *J Lab Cpds* 5: 168–172, 1969

8. WELCH MJ, LIFTON JF, SECK JA: Tracer studies with radioactive oxygen-15. Exchange between carbon dioxide and water. *J Phys Chem* 73: 3351–3356, 1969

9. TER-POGOSSIAN MM, EICHLING JO, DAVIS DO, et al: The determination of regional cerebral blood flow by means of water labeled with radioactive oxygen-15. *Radiology* 93: 31–40, 1969

10. EICHLING JO, RAICHLE ME, GRUBB RL, et al: Cerebral blood flow estimation employing the critical clearance of oxygen-15 labeled water. *Stroke*: to be published

11. TER-POGOSSIAN MM, EICHLING JO, DAVIS DO, et al: The measure in vivo of regional cerebral oxygen utilization by means of oxyhemoglobin labeled with radioactive oxygen-15. *J Clin Invest* 49: 381–391, 1970

12. GRUBB RL, RAICHLE ME, EICHLING JO, et al: Validation of the ^{15}O method for measuring regional oxygen utilization. Unpublished

13. EICHLING JO, RAICHLE ME, GRUBB RL, et al: In vivo determination of cerebral blood volume employing radioactive oxygen-15. *Circ Res*: to be published

14. RAICHLE ME, EICHLING JO, GADO M, et al: Cerebral blood volume in dementia. *Neurology* 24: 350, 1974

15. RAICHLE ME, GADO MH, EICHLING JO, et al: Cerebral hemodynamics and metabolism in pseudotumor cerebri. *Neurology* 24: 397, 1974

16. RAICHLE ME, EICHLING JO, GRUBB RL, et al: Cerebral blood volume in dementia. In *Intracranial Pressure*. II, Lundberg N, Ponten U, Brock M, eds, Berlin, Springer, 1975, pp 150–152

17. DITTMER DS, GREBE RM: *Handbook of Respiration*. Philadelphia, Saunders, 1958, p 5

18. O'BRIEN MD, VEALL N: Partition coefficients between various brain tumors and blood for ^{133}Xe. *Phys Med Biol* 19: 472–475, 1974

19. BUCKINGHAM PD, CLARK JC: Nitrogen-13 solutions for research studies in pulmonary physiology. *Int J Appl Radiat Isot* 23: 5–8, 1972

20. WELCH MJ: Production of active molecular nitrogen by the reaction of recoil ^{13}N. *Chem Comm* 1354–1355, 1968

21. CARTER CC, LIFTON JF, WELCH MJ: Organ uptake and blood pH and concentration effects of ammonia in dogs determined with ammonia labeled with ten-minute half-lived nitrogen-13. *Neurology* 23: 204–213, 1973

22. WELCH MJ, LIFTON JF: The fate of nitrogen-13 by the ^{12}C(d,n)^{13}N reaction in inorganic carbides. *J Am Chem Soc* 93: 3385–3388, 1971

23. TILBURY RS, DAHL JR, MONAHAN WG, et al: Production of nitrogen-13 labeled ammonia for medical use. *Radiochem Radioanal Lett* 8: 317–323, 1971

24. STRAATMANN MG, WELCH MJ: Enzymatic synthesis of nitrogen-13 labeled amino acids. *Radiat Res* 56: 48–56, 1973

25. LATHROP KA, HARPER PV, RICH BH, et al: Rapid incorporation of short-lived cyclotron-produced radionuclides into radiopharmaceuticals. In *Radiopharmaceuticals and Labelled Compounds*, vol 1, Vienna, IAEA, 1973, pp 471–481

26. EICHLING JO, GRUBB RL, RAICHLE ME, et al: Measurement of brain intracellular pH (pH$_i$) in vivo. Unpublished

27. RAICHLE ME, LARSON KB, PHELPS ME, et al: In vivo measurement of brain glucose transport and metabolism employing ^{11}C-glucose. *Am J Physiol*: to be published

28. STRAATMANN MG, HORTMANN AG, WELCH MJ: Production of 1-^{11}C-acetoacetic acid. *J Lab Cpds* 10: 175–179, 1974

29. RAICHLE ME, EICHLING JO, STRAATMANN MG, et al: Blood brain barrier permeability of ^{11}C-labeled alcohols and ^{15}O-labeled water. *Am J Physiol:* to be published

30. EICHLING JO, STRAATMANN MG, WELCH MJ, et al: Cerebral hematocrit of the rhesus monkey. *Circ Res*: to be published

31. WIELAND B: Development and evaluation of facilities for the efficient production of compounds labeled with carbon-11 and oxygen-15 at the Washington University Medical Cyclotron. Ph.D. Thesis, Ohio State University, December, 1973

32. MESSETER K, SIESJÖ BK: The intracellular pH in the brain in acute and sustained hypercapnia. *Acta Physiol Scand* 83: 210–219, 1970

33. RALL DP, OPPELT WW, PATLAK CS: Extracellular space of brain as determined by diffusion of insulin from the ventricular system. *Life Sci* 1: 43–48, 1962

34. ROOS A: Intracellular pH and intracellular buffering power of the cat brain. *Am J Physiol* 209: 1233–1246, 1965

35. LIFTON JF, WELCH MJ: Preparation of glucose labeled with 20-minute half-lived carbon-11. *Radiat Res* 45: 35–40, 1971

36. STRAATMANN MG, WELCH MJ: The liquid chromatographic purification of carbon-11 labeled glucose. *Int J Appl Radiat Isot* 24: 234–236, 1973

37. HORTON RW, MELDRUM BS, BACHELARD HS: Enzymic and cerebral metabolic effects of 2-deoxy-D-glucose. *J Neurochem* 21: 507–520, 1973

38. TAYLOR NF: The metabolism and enzymology of fluorocarbons and related compounds. In *Carbon-Fluorine Compounds. Chemistry, Biochemistry, and Biological Activities,* Elliot K, Birch J, eds, 1A Ciba Foundation Symposium, Amsterdam, Elsevier, 1972, pp 215–238

39. LAMBRECHT RM, WOLF AP: Cyclotron and short-lived halogen isotopes for radiopharmaceutical applications. In *Radiopharmaceuticals and Labelled Compounds,* vol 1, Vienna, IAEA, 1973, pp 275–290

40. ADAMSON J, FOSTER AB: 2-Deoxy-2-fluoro-D-glucose. *Chem Comm* 309–310, 1969

41. HOUSE HO, TROST BM: The chemistry of carbanions. X. The selective alkylation of unsymmetrical ketones. *J Org Chem* 30: 2502–2512, 1965

42. HOUSE HO, KRAMAR V: The chemistry of carbanions. V. The enolates derived from unsymmetrical ketones. *J Org Chem* 28: 3362–3379, 1963

43. RAICHLE ME, EICHLING JO, GRUBB RL: Brain permeability of water. *Arch Neurol* 30: 319–321, 1974

44. EICHLING JO, RAICHLE ME, GRUBB RL, et al: Evidence of the limitations of water as a freely diffusible tracer in the brain of the rhesus monkey. *Circ Res* 35: 358–364, 1974

45. EKLOF B, LASSEN NA, NILSSON L, et al: Regional cerebral blood flow in the rat measured by tissue sampling technique; a critical evaluation using four indicators ^{14}C-antipyrine, ^{14}C-ethanol, ^{3}H-water and ^{133}Xenon. *Acta Physiol Scand* 91: 1–10, 1974

46. CRONE C: The permeability of capillaries in various organs as determined by use of the indicator diffusion method. *Acta Physiol Scand* 58: 292–305, 1963

47. CHINARD FG, THAW CN, DELEA AC, et al: Intrarenal volumes of distribution and relative diffusion coefficients of monohydric alcohols. *Circ Res* 25: 343–357, 1969

48. STRAATMANN MG, WELCH MJ: A general method for labeling proteins with ^{11}C. *J Nucl Med* 16: 425–428, 1975

49. RICE RH, MEANS GE: Radioactive labeling of proteins in vitro. *J Biol Chem* 246: 831–832, 1971

50. CHRISTMAN D, CRAWFORD EJ, FRIEDKIN M, et al: Detection of DNA synthesis in intact organisms with positron-emitting methyl-^{11}C-thymidine. *Proc Natl Acad Sci USA* 69: 988–992, 1972

51. VEALL N, MALLETT BL: Regional cerebral blood flow determined by xenon-133 inhalation and external recording: the effect of arterial recirculation. *Clin Sci* 30: 353–369, 1966

52. OBRIST WO, THOMPSON HK, KING CH, et al: Determination of regional cerebral blood flow by inhalation of 133-xenon. *Circ Res* 20: 124–135, 1967

53. JONES T, BROWNELL GL, TER-PROGOSSIAN MM: "Equilibrium" images of short-lived radiopharmaceuticals for dynamic observations. *J Nucl Med* 15: 505, 1974

54. EFFROS RM, CHINARD FP: In-vitro pH of the extravascular space of the lung. *J Clin Invest* 48: 1983–1996, 1969

55. RAYNAUD C, TODD-POKROPEK AE, COMAR D, et al: A method for investigating regional variations of the cerebral uptake rate of ^{11}C labelled psychotropic drugs in man. In *Proceedings of Symposium on Dynamic Studies with Radioisotopes,* 1974, Oak Ridge, Tenn: to be published

Dynamic Time-Dependent Analysis and Static Three-Dimensional Imaging Procedures for Computer-Assisted CNS Studies

Thomas F. Budinger, Frank H. DeLand, Hector E. Duggan, John J. Bouz, Bernard Hoop, Jr., and William T. McLaughlin, and Paul M. Weber

D ynamic and static imaging of the brain using the scintillation camera and computers can be divided into four categories: (A) regional cerebral blood flow (rCBF) evaluation from counts versus time curves; (B) static image-enhancement procedures; (C) rCBF by parametric images; and (D) three-dimensional imaging from coded apertures or multiple camera views. This paper covers some of our experiences and results in these areas.

Quantitation of rCBF

Background and fundamental problems. The vascular blood volume of the brain is about 130 cc, and the circulation time through this vascular bed is about 8 sec. It is not well known how the flow or volume of distribution changes in disease states, but it is well known that even momentary cessation of brain blood perfusion causes loss of function. Thus there has been a continuing effort to derive some technique of brain bloodflow measurement for diagnostic as well as basic physiological studies of the hemodynamics of the normal brain. Our basic knowledge of brain blood flow comes from the work of Kety and Schmidt in 1948 (*1*) in which the Fick principle was used to derive the flow rate per unit mass (ml/100 gm/sec) for the whole brain from the observations of the disappearance of a diffusible tracer. This technique was improved for regional bloodflow assessment by the use of intracarotid injections of ^{85}Kr and ^{133}Xe and multiple probes or a scintillation camera to collect the washout data (*2–4*). The major drawback of these quantitative techniques for evaluating rCBF is the need for internal carotid artery injections. Thus other techniques using intravenous injections were sought.

It was hoped that with the advent of fast digital computers and scintillation cameras cerebral blood flow for cortical regions of the brain could be characterized by analysis of uptake-washout curves for nondiffusible tracers. One approach, first pursued by Oldendorf and Kitano (*5*), is to measure circulation time of an injected bolus by examining the count rate versus time curves representative of various regions of the brain. This idea is plagued by a fundamental problem: the flow, F, and mean transit time, $\bar{t}$, of a nondiffusible tracer through an organ are related to the organ blood volume, V, according to:

$$F = V/\bar{t}. \tag{1}$$

However, the circulation time as defined above is not simply related to the mean transit time, and the volume of the cerebral blood pool within the region of interest is generally unknown. Furthermore, it cannot be assumed that this volume is constant, since variations exceeding 100% between an engorged and a collapsed vascular system have been reported (*6*).

A second problem is the appearance of recirculating tracer before washout is complete. This type of nonlinear feedback is common to count rate versus time curves obtained with nondiffusible tracers and is particularly severe in the brain and heart. Such data do not easily lend themselves to analysis with tractable and applicable models of tracer kinetic behavior, particularly when the data are statistically poor. Most investigators have assumed that the downslope of the curve could be approximated by a single exponential function. For the brain, however, a more accurate approximation might be a gamma variate or other analytic function. A related problem is interference caused by the presence of overlying extracranial activity.

The third problem is difficulty in ascertaining the statistical significance of small differences in counts versus time curves. For example, suppose that a difference of 3 s.d. in counts recorded between two regions of interest is required for statistical significance. Then, if an average of 500 counts per region is recorded, as is the case for a region representing the middle cerebral artery on an anterior Towne's view, a 20% difference is required for detection of a lesion. This assumes perfect normalization of detector or scintillation camera response, which in itself is difficult to achieve to better than about 10%.

In spite of these difficulties, useful information can be derived from time-count rate curves obtained with external detectors by analysis of such parameters as: (A) transit time, measured between points of steepest ascent and descent of the uptake-washout curve; (B) time from the beginning to the peak of each curve; (C) slope of the washin curves; and (D) integral of the uptake curve up to the time that the earliest curve of a pair reaches maximum. Data of these sorts are usually best expressed as ratios of symmetrical regions of interest in the brain. These techniques do not give direct estimates of rCBF but establish circulation patterns related to disease conditions. The various methods are summarized in Fig. 4-1. The following sections describe the authors' experiences with these techniques. Intravenous injections of ^{99m}Tc-pertechnetate were used in all studies.

Transit time calculation. This method involves measuring the time duration between the points of inflection (maximum slope) in the uptake and washout portions of counts versus time curves (5). These two points represent the entrance and exit times for the most concentrated portion of the bolus. One way to objectively determine inflection points is to take the first derivative. However, as suggested by Fig. 4-1A, there are serious difficulties arising from curve irregularities, artifacts, and recirculation. This technique has not been found to be useful to us.

Uptake slope and time-to-peak activity. The slopes of the uptake curves for symmetrical regions of interest (Fig. 4-1B) or the times from injection to peak activity are simple parameters to determine and, when presented as ratios, give results commensurate with clinical observations. Unfortunately, the coefficient of variation is 20% for normals, and, when the deviations between right and left sides are greater than this value, the differences are seen equally well by simple inspection of sequential scintiphotos (7, 8). Differences in times of first appearance and times-to-peak activity are seldom of much diagnostic value (Table 4-1, columns A and B).

Integration of counts to the first maximum. Following the "Sapirstein principle" (9) that the initial distribution of a tracer ejected by the left ventricle reflects the fraction of cardiac output which that organ receives, Moses, et al (8) presented a technique for assessing rCBF using ^{99m}Tc-pertechnetate. The amount of activity accumulating in the region of interest during a period of about 12 sec after the injection (Fig. 4-1C) should be related to the fraction of cardiac output reaching the region of interest (10).

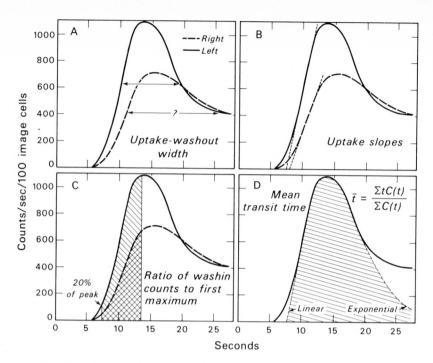

Fig. 4-1. Four methods of analyzing counts versus time curves to extract parameters comparing symmetrical regions of brain.

These methods were applied to a series of patients at Foothills Hospital using vertex and anterior views. The vertex view series included 73 patients with the following diagnoses: normal, carotid stenosis, supratentorial tumor, carotid occlusion, cerebral infarction, aneurysm, infratentorial tumor, subdural hematoma, craniotomy, and arteriovenous malformation. As many as ten regions of interest were examined on each patient. Results for the vertex view series are summarized in Table 4-1. Most (73%) of the mean values for the abnormal groups fell within ±2 s.d. of the normal values, indicating a generally poor separation between normals and abnormals. However, suggestive patterns were observed for supratentorial tumors, carotid occlusions, and infarctions, indicating that these groups do not come from the same normal pool.

The ratio of the total accumulated activity in symmetrical regions (vertex view) using a linear extrapolation for the washin portion of the counts versus time curve and a single exponential extrapolation of the washout portion was not found to be a sensitive criterion for the presence of abnormalities except perhaps for supratentorial tumors (Table 4-1, column E). Suggestive patterns were also observed for carotid occlusions and late cerebral infarctions; however, we could

TABLE 4-1. Mean Values for Five Pairs of Left/Right Regions of Vertex View of Head

Diagnosis	No. of patients	A Mean start time difference (sec) Mean	1 s.d.	B Mean peak time difference (sec) Mean	1 s.d.	C Mean ratio of counts to peak Mean	1 s.d.	D Mean time, t̄, difference (sec) Mean	1 s.d.	E Mean ratio of counts under extrapolated curve Mean	1 s.d.
Normal*	27	0.0	0.4	0.1	1.4	1.03	0.10	0.2	0.7	1.00	0.11
Stenosis†	9	0.2	0.5	-0.1	0.8	1.01	0.10	-0.2	0.8	1.03	0.16
Tumor supratentorial†	8	0.0	0.7	0.7	1.1	1.08	0.14	0.4	0.6	1.13	0.09
Carotid occlusion†	8	0.5	0.5	1.2	1.3	0.86	0.14	0.7	1.0	1.05	0.18
Infarction†	6	-0.2	0.7	0.1	0.7	1.02	0.16	0.9	0.7	1.13	0.12
Aneurysm†	5	0.0	0.2	0.0	0.8	0.99	0.08	0.0	0.8	0.99	0.04
Tumor infratentorial†	5	-0.1	0.3	-0.6	0.5	1.04	0.07	-0.1	0.8	1.02	0.04
Subdural hematoma†	2	0.0	—	0.7	—	0.86	—	0.6	—	0.96	—
Craniotomy†	2	0.4	—	0.8	—	0.92	—	1.6	—	1.21	—
AV malformation†	1	0.9	—	-0.6	—	0.92	—	-1.2	—	0.89	—

* Ratios listed are left/right side values. Time differences are left minus right side values.
† Ratios listed are abnormal/normal side values. Time differences are abnormal minus normal side values.

not conclude from data obtained in this series that these area/ratio techniques offer a significant improvement over dynamic flow scintiphotos.

A mean time parameter, $\bar{t}$, was calculated from:

$$\bar{t} = \frac{\Sigma_t t C(t)}{\Sigma_t C(t)} \tag{2}$$

where C(t) is the count at a particular time, t. Again, linear extrapolation was used on the ascending portion of the curve and exponential extrapolation on the descending portion. This mean time can be related to the mean transit time only for the case in which the tracer is introduced as an impulse and has uniform concentration over the entire vascular component (11). Such is clearly not the case here; thus it is important to distinguish the mean time, $\bar{t}$, from the mean transit time of Eq. 1. Differences in mean times for symmetrical regions in various pathological conditions are given for the vertex view in Table 4-1, column D. They were not remarkably greater than the normal variations.

In the anterior (frontal) projection series (263 patients), three bilateral regions of interest were used (12). They represented the carotid artery, middle cerebral artery, and anterior cerebral artery areas. The time segment for the accumulation phase was similar to that used by Moses, et al (8), but a venous phase time segment was also used in the analysis of data for the anterior and middle cerebral artery regions. The venous phase segment was that interval of time between the slowest peak and the beginning of the first plateau on the downslopes of the paired curves. Ratios of the smallest over the largest of the total counts in the paired time segments were calculated for the accumulation phase of the carotid artery regions and for the accumulation and venous phases of the middle cerebral and anterior cerebral artery areas. The normal ranges (mean ±2 s.d.) given in Table 4-2 compared well with our previous experience (12), with the results of studies done at Kaiser Permanente Hospital (unpublished), and with the results of Moses, et al (8).

The results of the venous phase analysis were found to be asymmetrical for arteriovenous malformations, cerebral vascular disease with delayed collateral circulation, and hypervascular tumors (12).

Benefits from counts versus time curves and derived quantitative parameters. Characterization of counts versus time curves for various regions of the brain after intravenous injection of radiotracers has not provided a significant new dimension in nuclear medicine studies of the brain. However, it has some important assets as an adjunct to rapid sequential cranial scintigraphy, including: (A) providing a quantitative criterion for normality in equivocal diagnostic cases and confidence in diagnostic impressions; (B) providing a means of quan-

TABLE 4-2. Normal Ranges (Means ± 2 s.d.) for Ratios of Symmetrical Regions for Anterior Projections (81 Patients)

Region	Range*
Internal carotid	0.80–1.0
Middle cerebral (accumulation)	0.83–1.0
Middle cerebral (venous)	0.80–1.0
Anterior cerebral (accumulation)	0.77–1.0
Anterior cerebral (venous)	0.74–1.0

* Ratio of lower to higher counts.

titatively evaluating return to normality after therapeutic measures, such as carotid artery surgery and radiotherapy; (c) aiding in the initial diagnosis by alerting the scintiphoto reviewer to questionable regions he has overlooked. It may also be useful for providing quantitative information regarding the collateral circulation in cerebral infarction, as described in the discussion of parametric images below.

Image Enhancement and Processing Techniques

In static brain imaging we are faced with the problem of interpreting a two-dimensional projection of a three-dimensional radionuclide distribution. Each point in the image is a summation of data from many small parts of the object volume, modified by attenuation and the point spread function of the imaging system. In addition, detector nonuniformities and scattered radiation contribute to further smear of the image. If the point spread function did not change markedly with distance from the collimator, the application of a single digital filter based on the particular collimator and detector response would give decided improvement in the images. However, this is not the case for imaging with conventional collimators. Moreover, the statistics of nuclear medicine imaging are photon limited; thus the statistical noise is multiplicative, which poses almost insurmountable problems compared to most image-processing problems in which the noise is additive, e.g., noise arising from electronic sources, etc. Some attempts have been made to improve images using thresholding, linear filters, and Wiener filters (13–19). Scintigrams with improved visual impact can be seen in the careful work of these authors, who also recognized the fundamental limitations of linear systems theory applied to nuclear medicine images. Recent results (unpublished) obtained with phantoms by some investigators have suggested that a small improvement in lesion detection capability could be achieved by some processing methods. Also, the routine automatic processing of images from dynamic flow studies has been found to be useful in a high workload nuclear medicine department (20). However, it has not yet been established whether there is a significant improvement in clinical diagnostic capability by static image processing or by other similar smoothing techniques (21, 22). Techniques such as contrast enhancement and thresholding convey results with improved visual impact but have not also been shown to improve diagnostic capability. These techniques are also easily effected by analog display systems and do not require the use of computers. Thus no great improvements have been found with the use of computerized image-processing techniques, and we cannot conclude that this area of effort will be of great value in the future.

Parametric or Functional Brain Images

A parametric image, also known as a "functional image," is a hybrid image showing the spatial distribution of some parameter or function such as the clearance rate, rate of flow, rate of uptake, ratio of ventilation to perfusion, etc. This type of image has been used by a number of investigators to show perfusion and clearance (23, 24). Parametric imaging of the brain is of limited use because of poor counting statistics. Nevertheless, there are some digital manipulations of dynamic flow data that take advantage of the quantitative aspects of count rate versus time curves from multiple regions of the brain and provide the clinician with a useful spatial image representing parameters from these curves.

N-MAX **image.** The N-MAX image shows the spatial distribution of elements in an image in which the maximum count rate during the 30-sec flow study falls within a specified interval (25). For example, in the vertex view shown in Fig. 4-2 a count rate between 10 and 15 cps is taken to represent cortical wash-through whereas a count rate between 25 and 30 cps represents the superior sagittal sinus. This image or a composite of images representing a series of intervals gives information about the relative blood pool size.

T-MAX **image.** The T-MAX image shows the spatial distribution of elements in an image that reach their maximum count rate during various time intervals of the 30-sec flow study (25). For example, the maximum flow to the cerebral hemispheres occurs about 10–15 sec after intravenous injection of radionuclide. Thus if there is a significant delay, say from unilateral carotid occlusion, the image for the period 10–15 sec will show activity in only one hemisphere. If collateral circulation is present, say from the ophthalmic artery to the affected hemisphere, then the image during the normal brain washout time 20–25 sec after injection would show diminished activity in the good side and maximum activity in the side with carotid occlusion (Fig. 4-3). The presence or absence of this "flip-flop" phenomenon

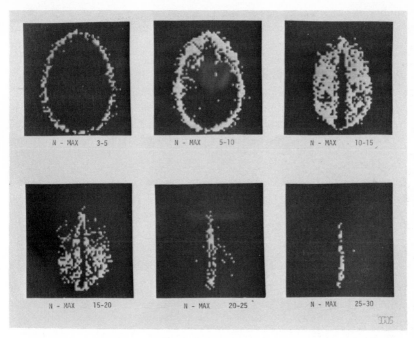

Fig. 4-2. N-MAX vertex images of normal subject showing image elements having maximum count rates during various intervals in 30-sec flow study. Numbers indicate time range in seconds.

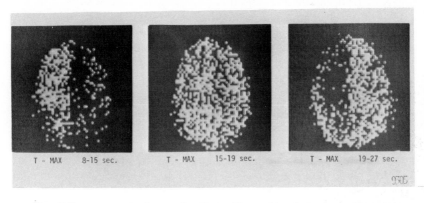

Fig. 4-3. T-MAX vertex image of subject with carotid occlusion and collateral circulation showing those image elements in which maximum count rate occurs during indicated time intervals in 30-sec flow study.

can be ascertained and quantitated by this technique as easily as with count rate versus time curves.

Equilibrium image. An equilibrium image is a scintigram obtained under steady-state conditions, during which time the rate at which radioactivity is appearing is equal to the rate at which it is disappearing from each point in the field of view. Acquisition of an equilibrium image implies administering the radiotracer at a constant rate to achieve equilibration (Chapter 3). While maintaining the pictorial qualities of conventional scintigrams, equilibrium images may also be used to extract quantitative dynamic information.

Examples of dynamic equilibrium images obtained on the Massachusetts General Hospital positron camera (26) are shown in Fig. 4-4. Left lateral views of the brain of a normal adult obtained during

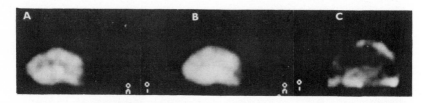

Fig. 4-4. Left lateral views of distribution of ^{15}O label in head 6–8 min after start of continuous inhalation of (A) O^{15}O, (B) CO^{15}O, and (C) C^{15}O.

constant inhalation of three different radioactive gases, O^{15}O, CO^{15}O, and C^{15}O (half-life, 2 min), are shown. Image data were collected starting at 6–8 min after inhalation of radioactive gas mixed into normal breathing air and supplied continuously to the subject at the rate of 1 mCi/breath. The inhaled gases, O^{15}O, CO^{15}O, and C^{15}O, label, respectively, oxyhemoglobin, water (via the rapid in vivo exchange of ^{15}O as CO$_2$ with H$_2$O), and carboxyhemoglobin (Chapter 3).

Figure 4-4A (O^{15}O) primarily depicts the distribution of labeled water produced by metabolism of the ^{15}O label transported to the cerebral tissue via oxyhemoglobin. Figure 4-4B (CO^{15}O) shows the distribution of labeled water transported to the brain as labeled H$_2$O. In this case the radiotracer is diffusible and is rapidly taken up in cerebral tissue; thus Fig. 4-4B represents, in part, distribution of cerebral blood flow. Figure 4-4C (C^{15}O) shows the brain blood pool distribution. That the ^{15}O activity in Fig. 4-4A and B is contained primarily in cerebral tissue can be seen by superimposing these images onto Fig. 4-4C, i.e., the sagittal sinus lies above the cerebral tissue volume. These examples of equilibrium images illustrate a potentially powerful approach to visualizing the distribution of cerebral function (blood volume, blood flow, and oxygen utilization) particularly with quantitative three-dimensional reconstruction techniques as described below and in Chapters 5 and 7.

Three-Dimensional Imaging

Coded apertures. We have investigated the use of two types of coded apertures: multiple pinholes (*27*) and a Fresnel zone plate (*28*). These techniques provide tomographic images of planes parallel to the plane of the detector. The resulting tomograms are not quantitative representations of the distribution at a particular depth because they present the in-focus distribution in the plane of interest superimposed on the out-of-focus distributions from contiguous planes. However, they do provide a means of clarifying and positioning suspicious areas of the static brain scan.

Pinhole tomography. Consider the arrangement shown in Fig. 4-5, in which a pinhole collimator is attached to a scintillation camera.

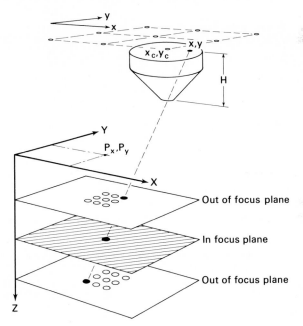

Fig. 4-5. Schematic of tomographic method employing multiple images from camera with successive displacements of patient relative to pinhole collimator.

The camera is moved to 36 positions separated by 2 cm in a matrix of 6 × 6 elements. Tomographic image slices can be prepared by reconstruction from these 36 images and assuming all activity exists at a particular depth. This gives the usual tomogram in which the activity in the reconstructed plane appears in focus but superimposed on the blurred activity from surrounding planes. The pinhole imaging geometry comprises two similar triangles in which the position of the image, x, y, is related to the position of a point source at X, Y in the object plane as:

$$X = -Z(x - x_c)/H; \quad Y = -Z(y - y_c)/H \tag{3}$$

where Z is the distance from pinhole to the object plane, H is the distance from the pinhole to the crystal, and x_c and y_c are at the center of the image plane. Here we have assumed that the center of the image and object planes and the pinhole are aligned on a common vertical axis. If the camera and pinhole collimator are displaced by P_x, P_y relative to the object plane, then Eq. 3 becomes:

$$X = -(Z/H) (x - x_c) - P_x \tag{4}$$

$$Y = -(Z/H) (y - y_c) - P_y. \tag{5}$$

Thus, for a point source located at a distance Z from the pinhole the tomographic slice for the plane at this depth can be calculated by computing X, Y for that value of Z and for each of many images taken at various displacements P_x, P_y from a reference center.

Thus if Eqs. 4 and 5 are repetitively applied to the picture elements for each of the displaced images, activity in a particular Z plane will appear in focus while activity in adjacent planes will be superimposed but out of focus. Figure 4-6 shows the results of a digitally reconstructed pinhole tomograph of a phantom containing ^{99m}Tc and a cold defect (27). The reconstruction time on the HP-5407 computer system at Donner Laboratory was 4 min for each plane.

As emphasized above, this technique does not give quantitative results. It is possible to calculate the contribution of the out-of-focus planes to the image by iterative techniques. This is not a simple problem and requires correction for attenuation; nevertheless, it could improve the results.

Another pinhole technique uses a multiple random pinhole distribution and gives similar results without the need for 36 separate images (29).

Digital reconstruction of Fresnel zone plate images. Fresnel zone plate imaging was first advocated for nuclear medicine imaging because of its potential for higher sensitivity gamma ray detection than can be obtained with the conventional pinhole or parallel-hole collimators (30, 31). It was argued that, because the geometrical efficiency of this and other coded aperture schemes was perhaps 1,000 or more times greater than that obtained with conventional collimators, a significant improvement in counting statistics would be realized. A more complete analysis now shows that there is not a great advantage in terms of signal-to-noise ratio with these techniques (28, 32). However, there remains a tomographic potential for these methods, and

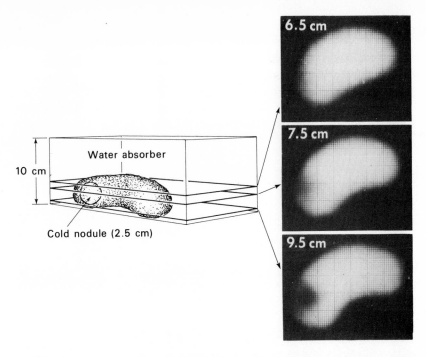

Fig. 4-6. Digitally reconstructed pinhole tomograph of phantom containing [99mTc] and cold defect. (Reprinted with permission from Ref. 27.)

we have devised a technique for digital reconstruction of the tomographic planes as follows.

First, the zone plate is placed between the object and the scintillation camera to form a coded shadowgram of the object. This image is digitized into a 64×64 matrix and then a phase shift is applied to each image element, $H(x,y)$, in the digitized shadowgram. The phase shift is a function of the zone plate parameters and of the distance between the object and the zone plate, and is given by:

$$H'(x,y) = H(x,y) \exp\{i\pi(x^2 + y^2)/R_1^2\} \tag{6}$$

where:

$$R_1 = R_0 \left\{1 + \frac{S_2}{S_1}\right\}. \tag{7}$$

R_0 is the radius of the first zone of the zone plate, S_1 is the distance from the object plane to the zone plate, and S_2 is the distance between the zone plate and the camera. A Fourier transformation is then applied to the resulting phase-shifted shadowgram to give the complex amplitude that, when squared, gives the image. The complete algorithm is thus:

$$I(x,y) = \mathscr{F}_2\left[H(x,y)\ \exp\!\left(\frac{i\pi(x^2 + y^2)}{R_1{}^2}\right)\right] \qquad (8)$$

where $\mathscr{F}_2$ denotes a two-dimensional spatial Fourier transform. An individual plane is reconstructed in approximately 27 sec on the HP-5407 computer at Donner Laboratory.

This method gives results that are not noticeably better than those of simple pinhole tomography. The tomographic capability is illustrated by Fig. 4-7.

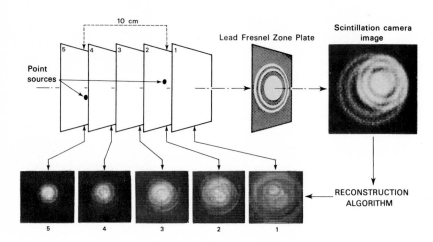

Fig. 4-7. Reconstruction of Fresnel zone plate images of two point sources. (Reprinted with permission from Ref. 28.)

Three-dimensional reconstruction techniques. As noted earlier, it is difficult to extract quantitative information from single views even with the application of tomographic techniques. This is one of the fundamental limitations in brain imaging and rCBF evaluation by conventional techniques. The three-dimensional distribution of a radiotracer in a patient can be determined by manipulation of digitized images from multiple scintillation camera views, to be described here (*33, 34*), or by the use of coincidence detection of positron annihilation photons, as described in Chapter 7.

The patient is rotated in 10-deg increments on a stool in front of an Anger scintillation camera (Fig. 4-8). The camera is equipped with a parallel-hole extended collimator constructed at Donner Laboratory. The collimator consists of 0.2-mm wall-thickness lead tubes, 12.7 cm long, which are stacked in close-packed hexagonal array. The purpose of the extension is to accommodate the shoulder and allow the patient's head to be as close to the collimator as possible.

Data are collected in 36 image frames of 64×64 elements using

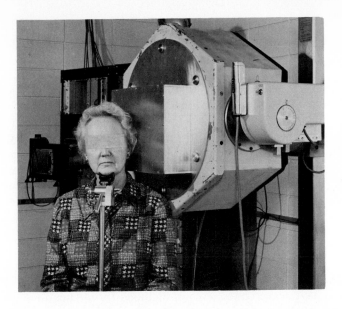

Fig. 4-8. Method of rotating patient in front of scintillation camera on stool fitted with chin holder to steady head. (Reprinted with permission from Ref. 33.)

the Hewlett-Packard HP-5407 computer system. Usually 50,000–100,000 counts/frame are collected in 30 sec in each view. The image elements are spaced at approximately 4-mm intervals.

An individual plane is reconstructed by selecting three rows of data from each of the 36 frames and using these as one-dimensional projections for reconstruction of a transverse section through the brain. The simplest reconstruction method is called back projection and is similar to that first used by Kuhl and Edwards in transverse section scanning (35). The simple superposition of a set of lines representing activity detected at various angles results in a blurring of the desired image no matter how many projection angles are observed (see Fig. 8-5).

Most reconstruction algorithms are attempts to deconvolute the true image from a back projection. Iterative techniques such as ART (arithmetic reconstruction technique) and the least-squares iterative technique solve for the best estimate of activity or count rate for an element $A(i,j)$ in a transverse section by minimizing the difference between the measured counts $P_{k(\theta)}$ and a value $R_{k(\theta)}$ estimated from an assumed transverse section distribution. Here k represents the kth measurement in a linear profile obtained at a projection angle θ. This assumed distribution might be an average value for each picture element $A(i,j)$, or the estimated distribution after an iteration wherein the estimated value $R_{k(\theta)}$ is

$$R_{k(\theta)} = \Sigma f_{ij}{}^{\theta,k} A(i,j). \qquad (9)$$

Here $f_{ij}{}^{\theta,k}$ is a weighting factor incorporating attenuation and the fractional intersection of a projection ray with the picture element of the transverse section being reconstructed.

One method of attenuation correction is performed as follows (Fig. 4-9). First, 36 views are obtained and 18 geometric mean projections are formed by taking the square root of the product of counts recorded in opposing (conjugate) views. Next, five iterations are done using the iterative least-squares algorithm, where $f_{ij}{}^{\theta}$ is set equal to 1.0, to determine the boundary of the object. The distance from each picture element to the boundary is determined for each angle θ, and the corresponding attenuation factor $f_{ij}{}^{\theta}$ is calculated. These factors are stored in a buffer that requires 76K words of storage for a 46×46 reconstructed array; thus the attenuation routine is a problem for a large computer. The final image is obtained by 8–10 iterations using the calculated values of $f_{ij}{}^{\theta}$ for all 36 projections.

We have investigated several methods for attenuation correction and find the fixed attenuation coefficient method described above to be adequate for the head. For the thorax we use an alternative correction technique based on a determination of attenuation coefficients from transmission data obtained by rotating the subject in front of a 20-mCi ^{99m}Tc source. These data are used to reconstruct a transverse section of attenuation coefficients using the iterative techniques or Fourier algorithms discussed below.

Fourier transform techniques for effecting a deconvolution of the true image arise from one of the following relations:

$$\text{True} = \mathscr{F}_2{}^{-1} |R| \mathscr{F}_2 \{\text{back projection}\} \qquad (10)$$
$$\text{True} = \mathscr{F}_2{}^{-1} \{\mathscr{F}_1 \text{ (projections)} * \delta(\theta,r)\} \qquad (11)$$
$$\text{True} = \text{back projection} \{\mathscr{F}_1{}^{-1} (|R| \mathscr{F}_1 \text{ (projections)})\} \qquad (12)$$

where $\mathscr{F}_n$ denotes an n-space Fourier transform, $\delta(\theta,r)$ is the delta function mapping the position of the Fourier coefficients from the projection data into the two-dimensional array, and $|R|$ is the spatial frequency. The method of Eq. 11 has been explored by others with phantoms (36). Our method uses Eq. 12, which is basically the technique used by Chesler with the positron camera (37). Thus each projection is modified by multiplying the Fourier transform of the projection by the spatial frequency radius. We then perform the inverse transform and back-project these modified projections. This procedure is about ten times faster than the iterative least-squares technique, and a cross section is reconstructed in 30 sec on the HP-5407 computer system.

Examples of clinical studies employing transverse section reconstructions are shown in Figs. 4-10 and 4-11. An abnormal accumula-

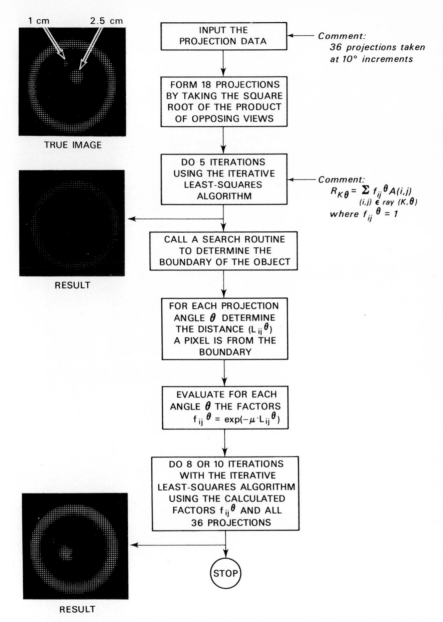

1 cm   2.5 cm

TRUE IMAGE

RESULT

RESULT

INPUT THE
PROJECTION DATA

Comment:
36 projections taken
at 10° increments

FORM 18 PROJECTIONS
BY TAKING THE SQUARE
ROOT OF THE PRODUCT
OF OPPOSING VIEWS

DO 5 ITERATIONS
USING THE ITERATIVE
LEAST-SQUARES
ALGORITHM

Comment:
$R_{K\theta} = \sum\limits_{(i,j) \,\epsilon\, ray \,(K,\theta)} f_{ij}{}^{\theta} A(i,j)$
where $f_{ij}{}^{\theta} = 1$

CALL A SEARCH ROUTINE
TO DETERMINE THE
BOUNDARY OF THE OBJECT

FOR EACH PROJECTION
ANGLE θ DETERMINE
THE DISTANCE $(L_{ij}{}^{\theta})$
A PIXEL IS FROM THE
BOUNDARY

EVALUATE FOR EACH
ANGLE θ THE FACTORS
$f_{ij}{}^{\theta} = \exp(-\mu \cdot L_{ij}{}^{\theta})$

DO 8 OR 10 ITERATIONS
WITH THE ITERATIVE
LEAST-SQUARES ALGORITHM
USING THE CALCULATED
FACTORS $f_{ij}{}^{\theta}$ AND ALL
36 PROJECTIONS

STOP

Fig. 4-9. Technique for applying attenuation correction with iterative least-squares algorithm.

tion of ^{99m}Tc-pertechnetate in the parietal-occipital region of a 50-year-old patient with brain tumors is shown in the transverse section images in Fig. 4-10. Figure 4-11 shows the results obtained on a 14-year-old patient, in which 36 images were acquired 6 hr after injection of 8 mCi of ^{99m}Tc-pertechnetate. Only about 10,000 counts were recorded in each view.

In general, the results obtained with ^{99m}Tc-pertechnetate for brain pathology indicate this method gives valuable clinical information, but at the present time emission reconstruction techniques take five times longer and provide far less resolution of anatomic detail than does CTT scanning.

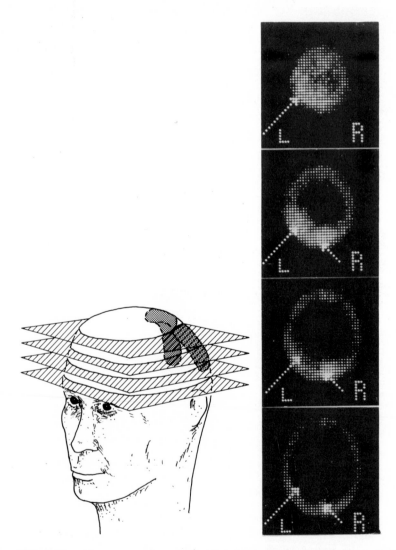

Fig. 4-10. Transverse section emission images of parietal-occipital tumors in 50-year-old patient.

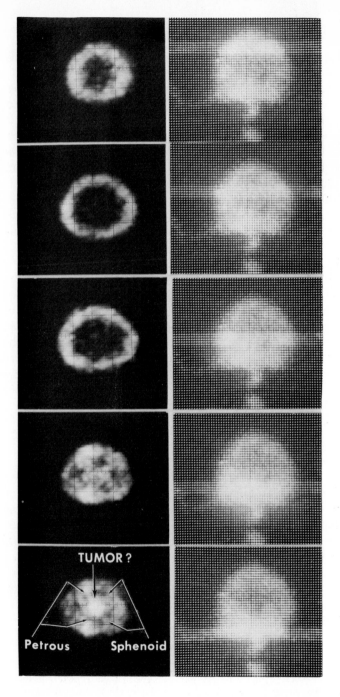

Fig. 4-11. Transverse section emission images (left) for sections shown in anterior view (right) from 14-year-old patient 6 hr after injection of 8 mCi ^{99m}Tc-pertechnetate. Activity is in region of chiasmatic cistern.

Conclusions

The use of computer techniques in nuclear medicine imaging of the brain began with the simple display of images and counts versus time curves reflecting the uptake and washout of tracers through the brain. Many problems relating to camera speed and data processing system speed (deadtime) have been overcome; yet, because of difficulties in the analysis of projections of three-dimensional distributions onto a two-dimensional plane, poor statistics, and the inability to define the volume of distribution for which the transit of tracer is being measured, computer manipulations have given results that fall short of expectations. Nevertheless, they provide a useful adjunct to the examination of sequential images from dynamic cerebral bloodflow studies and give the clinician some confidence in his diagnostic impressions.

Two-dimensional image-processing techniques have not proved to be of importance in diagnostic nuclear medicine primarily because the radionuclide distribution represents a three-dimensional problem. More recent developments in three-dimensional reconstruction from multiple views or multiple detectors promise to overcome the major limitations in previous work with digital computers. These techniques are now in clinical use for static imaging; however, speed limitations have prevented application to dynamic imaging. The future development of these methods will require innovations in patient positioning and multiple-view devices for either single-gamma or positron annihilation detection.

Acknowledgments

This work was done with financial support from the U.S. Atomic Energy Commission, the U.S. National Institutes of Health, and the Canadian Government. Associates who have contributed to this work are Hal Anger, Grant Gullberg, John Harpootlian, Burns MacDonald, Lucien Mathieu, James McRae, Brian Moyer, and Marcy Wales at Donner Laboratory and the Lawrence Berkeley Laboratory, Berkeley, Calif.; Myron Pollycove, San Francisco General Hospital, San Francisco, Calif.; and Dorothy Price, Santa Clara County Hospital, San Jose, Calif.

References

1. KETY SS, SCHMIDT CF: The nitrous oxide method for determination of cerebral blood flow in man: theory, procedure, and normal values. *J Clin Invest* 27: 476, 1948

2. GLASS HI, HARPER AM: Measurement of regional blood flow in cerebral cortex of man through intact skull. *Br Med J* 1: 593, 1963

3. LASSEN NA, HOEDT-RASMUSSEN K: Human cerebral blood flow measured by two inert gas techniques; comparison of the Kety-Schmidt method and the intra-arterial injection method. *Circ Res* 19: 681–694, 1966

4. PAULSON OB, CRONQVIST S, RISBERG J, et al: Regional cerebral blood flow: a comparison of 8-detector and 16-detector instrumentation. *J Nucl Med* 10: 164, 1969

5. OLDENDORF WH, KITANO M: Radioisotope measurement of brain blood turnover time as a clinical index of brain circulation. *J Nucl Med* 8: 570–587, 1967

6. HOEDT-RASMUSSEN K, SKINHOJ E, PAULSON O, et al: Regional cerebral blood flow in acute apoplexy with a demonstration of local hyperemia; the "luxury perfusion syndrome" of brain tissue. *Arch Neurol* 17: 271–279, 1967

7. FISH MB, POLLYCOVE M, O'REILLY S, et al: Vascular characterization of brain lesions by rapid sequential cranial scintiphotography. *J Nucl Med* 9: 249–259, 1968

8. MOSES DC, NATARAJAN TK, PREVIOSI TJ, et al: Quantitative cerebral circulation studies with sodium pertechnetate. *J Nucl Med* 14: 142–148, 1973

9. SAPIRSTEIN LA: Measurement of the cephalic and cerebral blood flow fractions of the cardiac output in man. *J Clin Invest* 4: 1429, 1962

10. WAGNER HN: Nuclear tracer studies of the cerebral circulation. *Hosp Prac* 8: 152–159, 1973

11. ZIERLER KL: Equations for measuring blood flow by external monitoring of radioisotopes. *Circ Res* 16: 309–321, 1965

12. McLAUGHLIN WT, PRICE DD, BUTLER T, et al: An update of the computer analysis of cephaloangioscintigraphy data. In *Proceedings of the Fifth Symposium of the Sharing of Computer Programs and Technoloy in Nuclear Medicine,* Salt Lake City, Utah, USAEC Report, CONF-750124, 1975, pp 138–154

13. BENDER MA, BLAU M: Data presentation in radioisotope scanning: contrast enhancement. In *Progress in Medical Radioisotope Scanning,* Kniseley RM, Andrews GA, Harris CC, eds, Oak Ridge, Tenn, USAEC, 1962, pp 105–110

14. GUSTAFFSON T, TODD-POKROPEK AE: Filters with variable shape in radioisotope image processing. Proceedings of a symposium: *The Data Processing and Data Handling of Radioisotope Scans,* Hanover, 1971: to be published

15. IINUMA TA: Image enhancement by the iterative approximation method. In *Quantitative Organ Visualization in Nuclear Medicine,* Kenny PJ, Smith EM, eds, Coral Gables, Fla, University of Miami Press, 1971, pp 549–580

16. KIRCH DL, BROWN DW: Recent advances in digital processing static and dynamic scintigraphic data. In *Proceedings of the Second Symposium on Sharing of Computer Programs and Technology in Nuclear Medicine,* Oak Ridge, Tenn, USAEC Report, CONF-720430, 1972, pp 27–54

17. LORENZ WJ, GEORGI P, MEDER HG, et al: Interactive processing and displaying of digital scintigrams. In *Medical Radioisotope Scintigraphy,* vol 1, Vienna, IAEA, 1972, pp 613–633

18. METZ CE: A mathematical investigation of radioisotope scan image processing. Ph.D. thesis, University of Pennsylvania, 1969

19. BUDINGER TF: Clinical and research quantitative nuclear medicine system. In *Medical Radioisotope Scintigraphy,* vol 1, IAEA, Vienna, 1972, pp 501–555

20. O'REILLY RJ, COOPER REM, RONAI PM: Automatic computer analysis of digital dynamic radionuclide studies of the cerebral circulation. *J Nucl Med* 13: 658–666, 1972

21. KUHL DE, SANDERS TD, EDWARDS RQ, et al: Failure to improve observer performance with scan smoothing. *J Nucl Med* 13: 752–757, 1972

22. METZ CE, GOODENOUGH DJ: On failure to improve observer performance with scan smoothing: A rebuttal. *J Nucl Med* 14: 873–876, 1973

23. KAIHARA S, NATARAJAN TK, WAGNER HN, et al: Construction of a functional image from regional rate constants. *J Nucl Med* 10: 347, 1969

24. MacIntyre WJ, Inkley SR: Functional lung scanning with [133]Xe. *J Nucl Med* 10: 355, 1969

25. DeLand FH, Bell PR, Fisher D: Pictorial display of quantitative temporal relationship of cerebral blood flow. Presented at 15th annual meeting of Southeastern Chapter, Society of Nuclear Medicine, St. Petersburg, Fla, 1974

26. Brownell GL, Burnham CA, Wilensky S, et al: New developments in positron scintigraphy and the application of cyclotron-produced positron emitters. In *Medical Radioisotope Scintigraphy,* vol 1, Vienna, IAEA, 1968, pp 163–176

27. Mathieu L, Budinger TF: Pinhole digital tomography. In *Proceedings of the First World Congress of Nuclear Medicine.* Tokyo, World Federation of Nuclear Medicine and Biology, 1974, pp 1264–1266

28. Budinger TF, Macdonald B: Reconstruction of the Fresnel-coded gamma camera image by digital computer. *J Nucl Med* 16: 309–313, 1975

29. Chang LT, Kaplan SN, Macdonald B, et al: A method of tomographic imaging using a multiple pinhole-coded aperture. *J Nucl Med* 15: 1063–1065, 1974

30. Barrett HH: Fresnel zone plate imaging in nuclear medicine. *J Nucl Med* 13: 382–385, 1972

31. Rogers WL, Han KS, Jones LW, et al: Application of a Fresnel zone plate to gamma-ray imaging. *J Nucl Med* 13: 612–615, 1972

32. Barrett HH, DeMeester GD: Quantum noise in Fresnel zone plate imaging. *Appl Opt* 13: 1100–1109, 1974

33. Budinger TF, Gullberg GT: Three-dimensional reconstruction in nuclear medicine emission imaging. *IEEE Trans Nucl Sci* NS-21: 2–20, 1974

34. Gordon R, Herman GT: Three-dimensional reconstruction from projections: a review of algorithms. *Int Rev Cytol* 38: 111–151, 1974

35. Kuhl DE, Edwards RQ: Image separation radioisotope scanning. *Radiology* 80: 653–661, 1963

36. Kay DB, Keyes JW Jr, Simon W: Radionuclide tomographic image reconstruction using Fourier transform techniques. *J Nucl Med* 15: 981–986, 1974

37. Chesler DA: Positron tomography and three-dimensional reconstruction technique. In *Tomographic Imaging in Nuclear Medicine,* Freedman GS, ed, New York, Society of Nuclear Medicine, 1972, pp 176–183

Chapter **5**

Computerized Emission Transaxial Tomography and Determination of Local Brain Function

David E. Kuhl, Abass Alavi, Martin Reivich,
Roy Q. Edwards, Craig A. Fenton,
and Robert A. Zimmerman

For the past several years we have employed computerized radio-nuclide transaxial tomographic scanning techniques for emission imaging of radionuclides in the brain (*1–3*). We have found the technique to be useful for the detection and separation of lesions, especially near the base of the brain. In addition, the technique shows promise as a method of quantitating radionuclide distributions in the brain for quantitative analysis of physiological parameters on a regional basis.

In concept, radionuclide and transmission transaxial scanning techniques (*4–6*; Chapter 8) have many similarities. However, they provide quite different and perhaps complementary types of information. Transmission techniques delineate attenuation differences in a cross section of the brain and seem best suited for the study of brain anatomy whereas emission techniques demonstrate the distribution of injected radiopharmaceuticals and are perhaps most useful for the study of brain function.

In this chapter we describe some comparative results obtained on patients by transmission and emission transaxial scanning techniques. We will also discuss application of quantitative aspects of the radionuclide technique for the measurement of local cerebral blood volume (LCBV).

Mark III Scanner

The results to be presented were obtained on our Mark III scanning system (7). The basic principles are illustrated in Fig. 5-1.

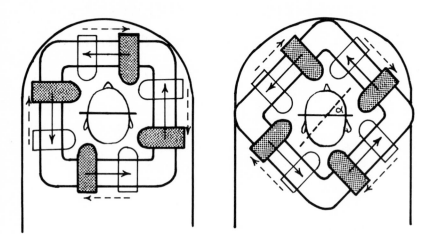

Fig. 5-1. Basic principles of transverse section scanning with Mark III scanner. Six linear scan passes are made with detector array rotated 15 deg between scans.

The scanner has four 2-in.-diam × ½-in.-thick NaI(Tl) detectors with focused collimators.

In a typical examination, the scanner first obtains conventional anterior, posterior, and lateral views, employing linear scan motion of the four detectors, while indexing the patient stepwise through the scanner between scan lines. The data are processed by an on-line computer to generate the scan images that are presented on a TV display system. The physician reviews the four scans and selects a scan line on the display for section scanning, using a knob on the display console that controls the movement of a blank TV scan line. The patient bed is moved automatically under computer control to position the detectors at the selected scan line. A transverse section scan is then obtained by performing a series of six linear scans at 15-deg increments around the head. For a patient injected with 10 mCi of ^{99m}Tc-pertechnetate these scans are completed in 3–5 min. The section scan data are processed by the computer using an orthogonal tangent correction (OTC) algorithm (8), and the final section image is presented on the TV display screen.

Comparison of Radionuclide and Transmission Scanning

We have only recently had a computerized transaxial transmission (CTT) system installed at our institution (EMI scanner with 160×160 matrix) and have done only a few comparison studies with our Mark III scanner and a conventional scintillation camera. However, a few of these early results will be presented to demonstrate the complementary nature of the radionuclide and transmission techniques.

Figure 5-2 shows conventional scintillation camera images ob-

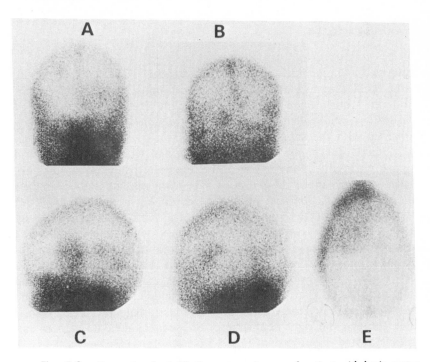

Fig. 5-2. Conventional scintillation camera images of patient with brain metastases after injection of ^{99m}Tc-pertechnetate. Multiple regions of increased uptake are apparent. (A) Anterior view; (B) posterior view; (C,D) lateral views; and (E) vertex view.

tained on a patient with metastatic lung carcinoma. Multiple lesions are apparent. The initial CTT scan (Fig. 5-3A) was also abnormal, but the lesions were more dramatic in the scan obtained after intravenous injection of contrast material (Fig. 5-3B). The com-

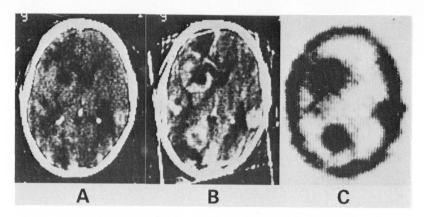

Fig. 5-3. Transmission and radionuclide section scans of same patient as in Fig. 5-2. (A) Conventional transmission scan; (B) transmission scan after intravenous injection of contrast material; and (C) radionuclide emission scan. Note clear separation of individual lesions in both transmission and radionuclide section scans and their superiority over camera vertex image in Fig. 5-2.

puterized radionuclide transaxial tomographic (CRTT) scan at the same level demonstrated the lesions with equal clarity (Fig. 5-3C). Both the transmission and the radionuclide scans clearly separated the lesions, and both were superior to the conventional vertex view obtained with the scintillation camera.

Figure 5-4 shows scans of a patient with an intracerebral hematoma involving the region of the internal capsule, posterior limb, and posterior part of the putamen. The conventional camera images showed a diffuse pattern of increased uptake in the left posterior temporal region (Fig. 5-4A and 5-4B). The CTT image dramatically defines the dense central hematoma (Fig. 5-4C). The radionuclide scan demonstrates a "doughnut" sign, probably representing increased uptake by infarcted tissue next to the hematoma.

Figure 5-5 shows a scintillation camera study of a patient with an infarction in the distribution of the right middle cerebral artery. The flow study was strikingly abnormal, demonstrating a prolonged transit time through the right hemisphere. Subsequent delayed camera images shown at the bottom of Fig. 5-5 were normal. However, the CTT scan (Fig. 5-6A) demonstrated a focus of reduced attenuation in the region of the right internal capsule with extension into the right frontal lobe. The CRTT scans (Fig. 5-6B and C) also demonstrated a minimal but definitely increased uptake of radionuclide in the same region.

This case illustrates reinforcement of diagnosis by complementary transmission and radionuclide data. It also shows that both radionuclide and transmission section scanning can demonstrate lesions that cannot be seen by conventional radionuclide imaging.

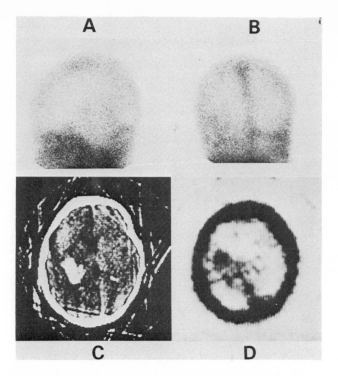

Fig. 5-4. Transmission and radionuclide images of patient with intracerebral hematoma. (A) Conventional ^{99m}Tc-pertechnetate lateral view with scintillation camera; (B) camera posterior view; (C) transmission section scan; and (D) emission section scan. Abnormality is seen on all four images but with greatest clarity on section scans. Radionuclide section scan demonstrates doughnut sign, probably representing infarcted tissue adjacent to hematoma.

Local Cerebral Blood Volume

Recent advances in the development of reconstruction algorithms for CRTT scanning have made it possible to obtain images in which the image density is linearly related to radionuclide concentration within the examined section (8–10). A digital representation of such an image can therefore be quantitatively related to radionuclide content. In our work we have employed the orthogonal tangent correction (OTC) algorithm and a correction mask to correct for attenuation (8). We estimate that we can predict radionuclide concentration within a 2-cm-diam area of a section to within 6% (s.d.) (Fig. 5-7).

We have employed quantitative radionuclide section scanning for the study of LCBV (11). Measurement of LCBV in patients would be useful for assessing cerebral hemodynamics. Changes in LCBV are known to occur in physiological states such as mentation (12) and

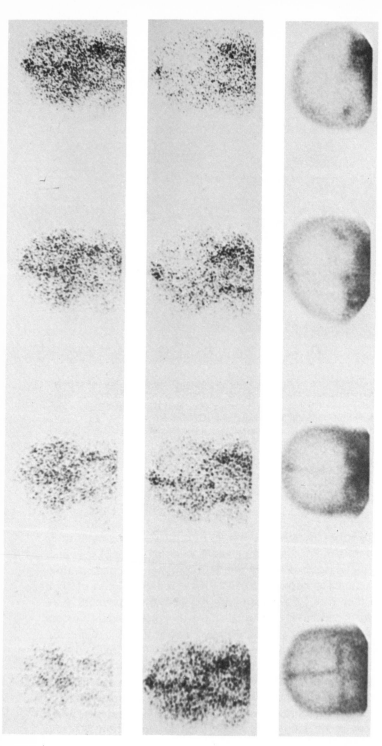

LPOST**R**   R**ANT**L   A**LT.LAT**P   P**RT.LAT**A

Fig. 5-5. Scintillation camera study of patient with infarction of right middle cerebral artery. Initial 99mTc-pertechnetate flow sequence (top two rows) is strikingly abnormal, demonstrating prolonged transit time through right hemisphere (left side of scintigrams). Subsequent delayed static images (bottom row) appear completely normal.

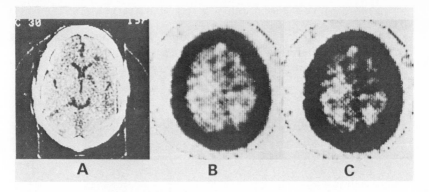

Fig. 5-6. Transmission and emission section scans of same patient as in Fig. 5-5. (A) Transmission scan demonstrating focal reduced attenuation in region of right internal capsule with extension into frontal lobe. (B,C) Emission scans showing increased uptake of radioactivity in same region.

sleep (*13*), with alteration of arterial CO_2 tension (*14*), and in pathological states such as increased intracranial pressure (*15*). However, accurate measurement of LCBV in vivo is difficult. Techniques employing external radionuclide counting are complicated by interference from radionuclide concentrations in the overlying scalp and cranium (*16*) and often require intra-arterial injections (see Chapter 3).

To avoid these problems we have developed a relatively noninvasive method for absolute measurement of LCBV in three dimensions throughout the brain. The method employs an injection of ^{99m}Tc-labeled red cells into a peripheral vein followed by CRTT scanning of the brain. A blood sample is taken during the scan and the concentration of activity in red cells and in plasma is determined. The digitally reconstructed scan image and the measured concentration of blood radioactivity are used to determine LCBV in ml blood/100 gm of brain tissue. The result is a two-dimensional map of LCBV for a cross section of the brain at a known level.

In a series of four baboons, we found good agreement between the section scan and the results from in vitro counting of brain samples. The coefficient of variation was 6.7% for calculations of brain activity concentrations and 8.1% for LCBV. The reproducibility of the scan method was estimated over a time period of several hours using an animal maintained in a steady state. The mean of the scan-determined LCBV values for a 2-cm square in the center of the brain was 3.22 ml blood/100 gm with a coefficient of variation of 6.5%.

In a series of five baboons, the following regression was obtained between LCBV at the center of the brain and P_aCO_2 (mm Hg) and mean arterial blood pressure (MABP):

$$LCBV = 2.88 + 0.049\ P_aCO_2 - 0.013\ MABP \qquad (1)$$

These results are in good agreement with some other results reported in the literature (Table 5-1).

Figure 5-8 shows the normalized regression planes for LCBV

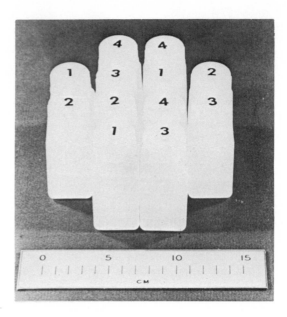

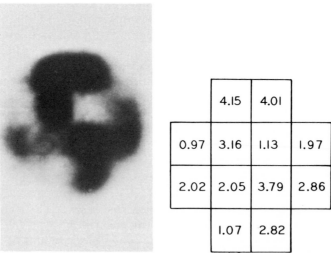

		4.15	4.01	
0.97	3.16	1.13	1.97
2.02	2.05	3.79	2.86
	1.07	2.82	

Fig. 5-7. Demonstration of accuracy of emission section scanning for predicting radioactive concentrations. Actual concentrations are labeled on top of vials (top). Calculated concentrations are indicated in diagram at bottom right. Picture at bottom left shows reconstructed image. Total of 1.5 million counts was collected.

TABLE 5-1. Response of LCBV Measured by Transaxial Emission Tomography to P_aCO_2 and MABP and Comparison to Previous Work

Animal	P_aCO_2 slope	MABP slope	References
Goat	0.043		Smith, et al (15)
Rhesus monkey	0.049		Phelps, et al (17)
Rhesus monkey		−0.015	Grubb, et al (18)
Baboon	0.049	−0.013	Present study

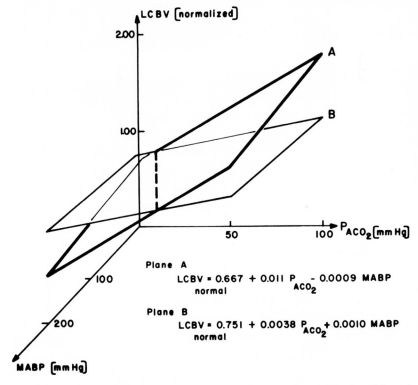

Plane A

$$LCBV_{normal} = 0.667 + 0.011\ P_{ACO_2} - 0.0009\ MABP$$

Plane B

$$LCBV_{normal} = 0.751 + 0.0038\ P_{ACO_2} + 0.0010\ MABP$$

Fig. 5-8. Regression planes for local cerebral blood volume (LCBV) vs. P_aCO_2 and mean arterial blood pressure (MABP). Plane A: Measured from reconstructed transverse section scan. Plane B: Measured from same external counting data, before reconstruction. (Reprinted with permission of the American Heart Association, Inc.; Ref. 11.)

determined from CRTT scans (A) and from counting data without reconstruction (B). Note the disparity in slopes. External counting without section reconstruction is an inaccurate indicator of LCBV because it does not discriminate against the effect of extracerebral circulation.

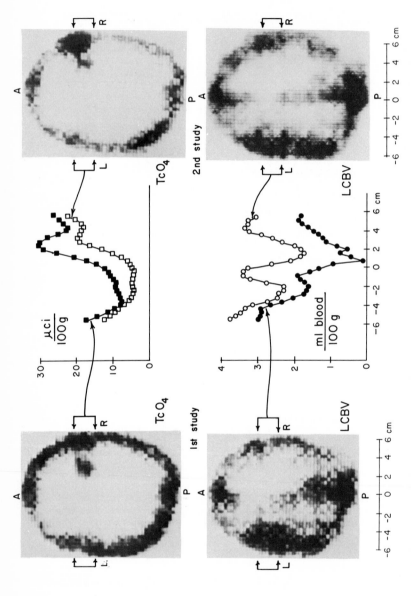

Fig. 5-9. Study of LCBV in patient with malignant glioma surrounded by edema. Top row shows data for ^{99m}Tc-labeled red blood cells. **Left:** Initial scans. **Right:** Scans taken 2 months later after steroid therapy. **Center:** Profiles of pertechnetate activity (top) or LCBV (bottom) across section images. Initially, LCBV is reduced in region of tumor because of compression of microcirculation by edema. After steroid therapy, LCBV returns toward normal. (Reprinted with permission of the American Heart Association, Inc.; Ref. 11.)

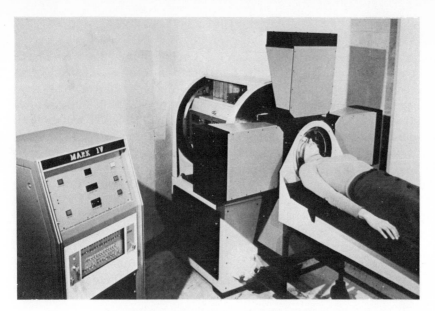

Fig. 5-10. Mark IV transverse section scanner.

In a preliminary study of patients, LCBV values ranged from 2 to 4 ml/100 gm depending on location, with higher values corresponding to regions of cerebral cortex. An example of an LCBV study on a patient with a malignant glioma is shown in Fig. 5-9.

Mark IV Scanner

Until recently the full utilization of CRTT scanning in our laboratory was hampered by the low sensitivity of the Mark III scanner. We have now completed and are testing the Mark IV transverse section imaging system, which was designed to be at least ten times more sensitive than the Mark III instrument. The device (Fig. 5-10) uses a continuously rotating set of four collimated NaI(Tl)-detector arrays. Each array is comprised of a linear arrangement of eight 3-in.-high × 1-in.-wide × 1-in.-thick detectors. As the detector arrays are rotated, data are collected continuously using 32 pulse height analyzers. Image reconstruction is accomplished at the same time with a virtual real-time processing and display system. Initially the instrument will be used primarily with ^{99m}Tc, but modifications are also planned to allow alternative use for coincidence counting of positron emitters.

Conclusions

Accurate knowledge of regional function in the brain would be of great value for the detection and localization of a wide variety of diseases and for assessment of patients under treatment. The management of patients would be greatly improved with a day-to-day knowledge of the status of blood flow, blood volume, metabolism, permeability, brain swelling, and other functions on a local basis throughout the brain. In the past this kind of information has not been available. Instead, function has usually been examined only for the organ as a whole and regional information has been restricted to morphology as determined by radiographic or radionuclide imaging studies. Three-dimensional radionuclide reconstruction imaging will become more important in the study of the brain, providing accurate measurement of radionuclide concentration within functional structural units of the brain. Measurement of local function with three-dimensional resolution throughout the brain and without the necessity for intracarotid injection of indicator could therefore provide a significant advance over presently available methods.

Acknowledgment

This work was supported in part by USPHS Research Grant 2R01 GM-16248, USAEC Contract AT(11-1)-3399, USPHS Program Project Grant 5P01NS-10930, and USPHS Research Career Development Award 5K03-HL-11,896 (Dr. Reivich).

References

1. KUHL DE, EDWARDS RQ: Image separation radioisotope scanning. *Radiology* 80: 653-662, 1963

2. KUHL DE, PITTS FW, SANDERS TP, et al: Transverse section and rectilinear brain scanning using ⁹⁹ᵐTc pertechnetate. *Radiology* 86: 822-829, 1966

3. KUHL DE, SANDERS TP: Characterizing brain lesions using transverse section scanning. *Radiology* 98: 317-328, 1971

4. KUHL DE, HALE J, EATON WL: Transmission scanning: a useful adjunct to conventional emission scanning for accurately keying isotope deposition to radiographic anatomy. *Radiology* 87: 278-284, 1966

5. HOUNSFIELD GN: Computerized transverse axial scanning (tomography): Part 1. Description of system. *Br J Radiol* 46: 1016-1022, 1973

6. AMBROSE J: Computerized transverse axial scanning (tomography): Part 2. Clinical application. *Br J Radiol* 46: 1023-1047, 1973

7. KUHL DE, EDWARDS RQ: The MARK III scanner: a compact device for multiple-view and section scanning of the brain. *Radiology* 96: 563-570, 1970

8. KUHL DE, EDWARDS RQ, RICCI AR, et al: Quantitative section scanning using orthogonal tangent correction. *J Nucl Med* 14: 196-200, 1973

9. Ter-Pogossian MM, Phelps ME, Hoffman EJ, et al: A positron-emission transaxial tomograph for nuclear imaging (PETT). *Radiology* 114: 89–98, 1975

10. Budinger TF, Gullberg GT: Three-dimensional reconstruction in nuclear medicine by iterative least-squares and Fourier transform techniques. USAEC Report LBL-2146, TIC-4500-R61, 1974

11. Kuhl DE, Reivich M, Alavi A, et al: Local cerebral blood volume determined by three-dimensional reconstruction of radionuclide scan data. *Cir Res* 36: 610–619, 1975

12. Risberg J, Ingvar DH: Regional changes in cerebral blood volume during mental activity. *Exp Brain Res* 5: 72–78, 1968

13. Risberg J, Gustavsson L, Ingvar DH: Regional cerebral blood volume during paradoxical sleep. In *Cerebral Blood Flow. Clinical and Experimental Results,* Brock M, Fieschi C, Ingvar DH, et al, eds, Berlin, Springer, 1969, pp 101–102

14. Smith AL, Neufeld G, Ominsky AJ, et al: Effect of arterial CO_2 tension on cerebral blood flow, mean transit time, and vascular volume. *J Appl Physiol* 31: 701–707, 1971

15. Langfitt TW, Weinstein JD, Kassell NF: Cerebral vasomotor paralysis produced by intracranial hypertension. *Neurology* 15: 662–641, 1965

16. Oldendorf WH, Lisaka Y: Interference of scalp and skull with external measurements of brain isotope content: Part 1. Isotope content of scalp and skull. *J Nucl Med* 10: 177–183, 1969

17. Phelps ME, Grubb RL, Ter-Pogossian MM: Correlation between $PaCO_2$ and regional cerebral blood volume by x-ray fluorescence. *J Appl Physiol* 35: 274–280, 1973

18. Grubb RL, Phelps ME, Raichle ME, et al: The effects of arterial blood pressure on the regional cerebral blood volume by x-ray fluorescence. *Stroke* 4: 390–399, 1973

Chapter 6

Tomographic Radionuclide Brain Imaging with the Anger Tomoscanner

Ernest W. Fordham and David A. Turner

We are currently evaluating the clinical performance of a commercial prototype of the tomographic rectilinear scanner described by H. O. Anger (1, 2). This is a dual-probe, rectilinear scanner
with 8-in.-diam detectors that generates tomographic images in 12
planes simultaneously during a single scan. In this report we will describe our preliminary observations on its application in brain imaging.

The quality of the tomographic images acquired with this instrument appears to be at least as good as that provided by the standard
Anger camera. However, the tomographic technique can provide
additional diagnostic information in some patients, and it therefore
may be employed as a special procedure in selected cases. In our
experience this technique has been particularly useful in the evaluation of the posterior fossa, the pituitary region, and the anterior
temporal area, and in the distinction between calvarial and intracranial lesions. The following case studies were selected as illustrative
material. All of these patients were studied with ^{99m}Tc-pertechnetate
(20 mCi), following oral administration of 1 gm NaClO$_4$. A total of
400,000 counts was obtained for the conventional Anger camera
images. In the tomoscanner series the planes were separated by
approximately 1-in. intervals and the most superficial planes are on
the left in all figures.

Radionuclide images obtained from a 62-year-old woman with

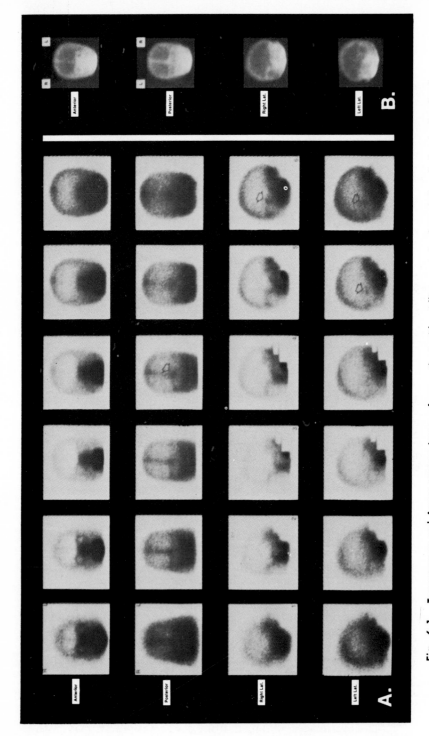

Fig. 6-1. Tomoscanner and Anger camera images from patient with midline posterior fossa lesion. Lesion is visualized (arrows) in tomoscanner series (A) but is indistinguishable from vascular structures in Anger camera images (B).

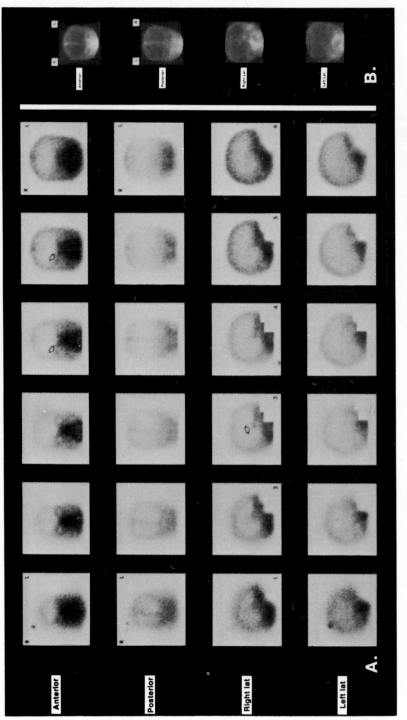

Fig. 6-2. Tomoscanner and Anger camera images from patient with lesion deep to right temporalis muscle. Lesion is visualized (arrows) in tomoscanner series (A) but is indistinguishable from temporalis activity in Anger camera images (B).

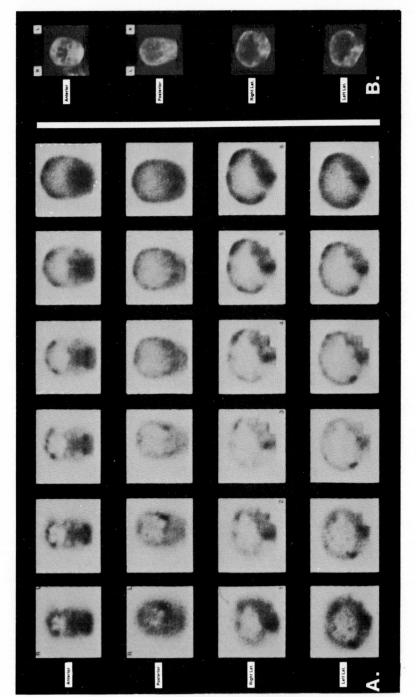

Fig. 6-3. Tomoscanner and Anger camera images from patient with multiple metastases to skull. Tomoscanner series (A) demonstrates superficial nature of lesions and normal distribution in brain, which is not clear from Anger camera images (B).

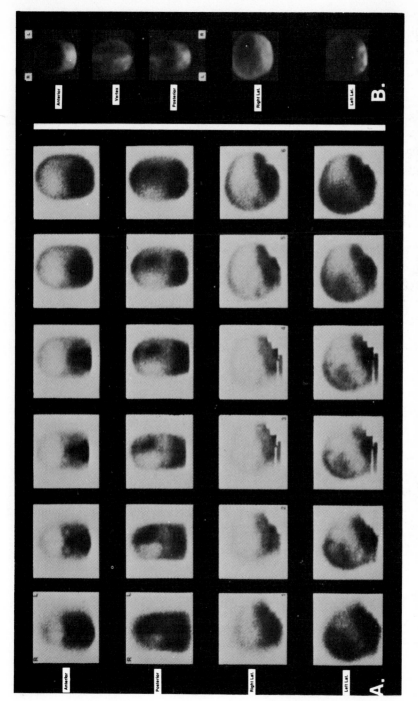

Fig. 6-4. Tomoscanner and Anger camera images from patient with intracerebral lesion underlying increased activity in a craniotomy defect. Lesion and defect are separated in tomoscanner series (A) but not in Anger camera images (B).

suspected metastatic breast cancer and symptoms referable to the posterior fossa are shown in Fig. 6-1. A computerized transaxial tomographic scan of this patient demonstrated enlarged lateral ventricles as the only abnormality. The Anger camera images were interpreted as normal. Tomographic scans demonstrated a discrete lesion in the midline of the anterior region of the posterior fossa, which, in contrast to the Anger camera images, could be clearly distinguished from the torcula and lateral sinuses.

Figure 6-2 illustrates radionuclide images obtained from a 54-year-old woman, 8 months after an incomplete abdominal perineal resection of a rectal carcinoma. The camera images show prominent activity in the right anterior temporal region but were interpreted as normal. The tomographic scans show a lesion lying deep to temporalis muscle in the right lateral views and also demonstrate the lesion in two sequences of the anterior views.

Images from a 60-year-old woman with known diffuse skeletal metastases from breast cancer are shown in Fig. 6-3. Multiple lesions are seen in the camera images. However, the tomographic images clearly demonstrate the superficial location of these lesions within the skull, and were useful in the exclusion of cerebral metastases.

Images from a 34-year-old woman, 6 months following craniotomy and removal of a metastatic melanoma from the left parietal lobe, are shown in Fig. 6-4. The camera images demonstrate increased activity over the left parietal region, which was attributed to the craniotomy defect. The tomographic images clearly show the superficial craniotomy defect as well as an underlying intracerebral lesion.

We have found that, in addition to providing valuable new information as illustrated in the above examples, the Anger tomoscanner is often helpful by more clearly defining lesions and thus increasing the degree of confidence in diagnoses obtained on the basis of conventional camera images. Furthermore, the technique seems practical since it requires only slightly more time than conventional Anger camera imaging. It can be used to eliminate the need for obtaining additional special views with the camera, and in a busy nuclear medicine service this would allow for more efficient scheduling and a smoother flow of patients, as well as providing a technique capable of acquiring important additional diagnostic information.

References

1. ANGER HO: *Fundamental Problems in Scanning,* Springfield, Ill, Charles C Thomas, 1968, p 195

2. ANGER HO: Multiplane tomographic scanner. In *Tomographic Imaging in Nuclear Medicine,* Freedman GS, ed, New York, Society of Nuclear Medicine, 1973, pp 1–18

Transaxial Emission Reconstruction Tomography: Coincidence Detection of Positron-Emitting Radionuclides

Michael E. Phelps, Edward J. Hoffman,
Nizar A. Mullani, and Michel M. Ter-Pogossian

The improvements that have been realized with computerized transaxial tomography (CTT) in radiographic transmission imaging (Chapter 8) are also possible in radionuclide imaging. Prior to the introduction of the EMI scanner, the general principle of transaxial reconstruction tomography had already been applied by Kuhl, Edwards, and coworkers (1–4) to cross-sectional imaging of radionuclide distributions in the brain (Chapter 5). Kuhl's system employed a series of rectilinear scans at discrete angles around the head with collimated scintillation detectors. Kuhl's approach has also been applied with some modifications by a number of other investigators (5–10). Still other investigators have described transaxial reconstruction tomography with the scintillation camera (11–14; Chapter 4). All of these reports have described single photon counting (SPC) systems. SPC refers to a system in which individual photons are counted without a requirement for time coincidence detection of multiple photons.

The technique to be described here employs annihilation coincidence detection (ACD) of positron-emitting radionuclides. ACD refers to the coincidence detection of two 511-keV photons emitted at

180 deg to each other following positron annihilation. Brownell, et al (*15, 16*) have successfully developed a camera for imaging positron-emitting radionuclides and Chesler (*17, 18*) has applied the system to transaxial tomographic imaging. Robertson, et al (*19*) used a ring of detectors operating in coincidence for tomographic imaging. Some of the advantages of ACD as compared to SPC systems have been described by these authors and by Cormack (*20*).

Some of the work to be presented here has also been described by Phelps, et al (*21*) and Ter-Pogossian, et al (*22*).

General Requirements and Criteria for CRTT

The objective of computerized radionuclide transaxial tomography (CRTT) is to generate an image showing the distribution of radioactivity in a cross-sectional slice of the object. Data for a CRTT image are obtained by performing linear scans at a series of discrete angles around the object (Fig. 7-1). Count rate profiles from the linear

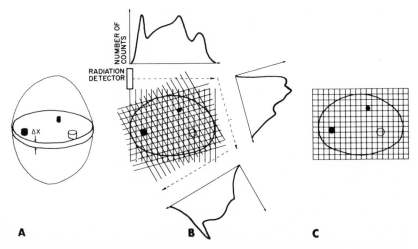

Fig. 7-1. Schematic representation of transaxial emission reconstruction tomography. (A) Slice of thickness Δx in object containing one "cold" and two "hot" defects. (B) Count rate profiles recorded from linear scans of same slice taken at different angles. (C) Mathematically reconstructed image of slice from many profiles as in (B). (Reprinted with permission from Ref. 21.)

scans serve as input data for a computer, which employs a mathematical algorithm to calculate the distribution of activity within the examined slice. Many of the considerations relating to the mathematical algorithm, the required number of linear and angular data points (sampling frequency), and full angle through which data should be taken are the same for the radionuclide case as they are for the transmission case and are discussed in detail in Chapter 8. In this section we will discuss special considerations pertaining to CRTT scanning.

Two assumptions of CRTT scanning are that the slice is a plane (thickness $\Delta x = 0$, Fig. 7-1) and that each detector reading corresponds to a linear sum of activity in a well-defined region across the examined slice. The first assumption reduces the reconstruction problem from three to two dimensions and thus activity variations in the vertical direction (thickness of slice) are represented as a part of the variations in the cross-sectional plane. This suggests that for optimum perception of three-dimensional objects, the thickness of the slice should be comparable to the scanning resolution within the cross section. The second assumption requires that the detection system have a constant resolution and sensitivity with depth so that each detector reading, Y, can be represented as a linear sum:

$$Y = k(A_1 + A_2 + A_3 + \ldots A_i) \tag{1}$$

where A_1 through A_i represent the activities in individual grid elements seen by the detector, and k is a sensitivity constant (counts per activity). Thus the detector collimation should exhibit constant resolution and counting sensitivity with depth, and methods of correcting for variations in sensitivity with depth caused by attenuation should be applied.

In the final reconstructed image each image element should represent, in a quantitative manner, the amount of activity in a small volume (e.g., a 1-cm cube) within the slice. This fact might raise serious questions about the usefulness of tomography in the photon-limited field of nuclear medicine, since it would appear that a long counting time would be required to determine accurately the amount of activity in such small volumes. By contrast, in conventional imaging with a scintillation camera or a scanner, the resolution in two dimensions may be small, but in the third dimension, depth, it is much larger. Each image element thus represents activity in a considerably larger volume than in CRTT imaging, and shorter imaging times would appear to be required. However, it must be remembered that, in attempting to resolve a small volume of activity by conventional two-dimensional imaging techniques, many of the counts arising from the large volume of activity in depth carry no useful information and are in fact only an added source of noise. Therefore, the two imaging techniques (conventional and CRTT) are comparable in terms of the volume of the tissue of interest to be measured. This does not necessarily mean that CRTT imaging will require shorter counting times than conventional imaging, since one of its aims is to produce images with greater detail, which therefore requires higher information densities. However, a well-designed CRTT system will generate statistically valid cross-sectional images in counting times of 1–2 min/slice as will be seen from examples to be presented later in this chapter. This is not too different from conventional imaging techniques.

Principles of Annihilation Coincidence Detection

In annihilation coincidence detection (ACD), events are recorded as valid only when two 511-keV photons from positron annihilation are recorded simultaneously in two opposing radiation detectors. Since the two 511-keV photons are emitted at 180 deg, this limits the field of view to a well-defined region between the two detectors (Fig. 7-2). This establishes an "electronic" collimation and eliminates the need for the conventional lead absorption-type collimators.

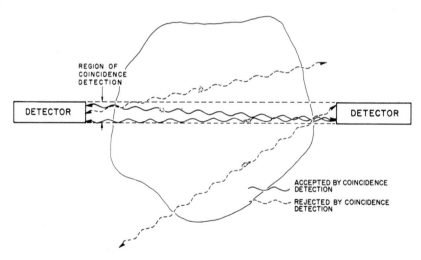

Fig. 7-2. Detection of annihilation coincidence photons. Events are accepted only when two 511-keV annihilation photons emitted at 180 deg strike two opposing detectors simultaneously. All other events are rejected. (Reprinted with permission from Ref. 21.)

Spatial resolution. The line spread functions (LSFs) for a positron-emitting line source (^{64}Cu) in a 24-cm-thick water phantom are shown in Fig. 7-3A. These measurements were taken with two 5-cm-diam × 5-cm-thick NaI(Tl) detectors connected in coincidence and separated by a distance of 54 cm. Single-channel analyzers were set to accept only photopeak events. The 5-cm-diam detectors were shielded with a 2.5-cm-thick lead plate with a 2.5-cm straight bore hole over the center of each detector. The lead shield was added to

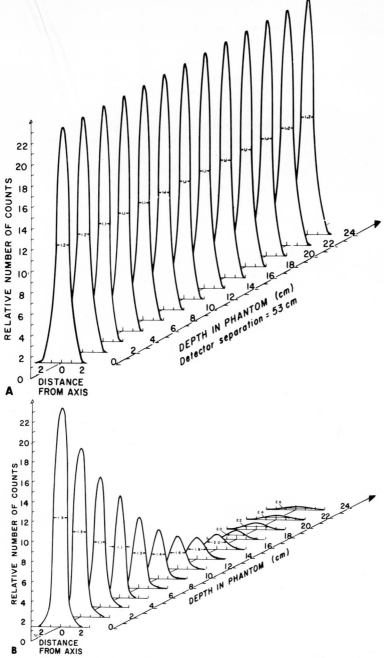

Fig. 7-3. (A) LSF for annihilation coincidence detection, ACD (^{64}Cu), employing 5-cm-diam × 5-cm-thick NaI(Tl) detectors. Lead shields (2.5 cm thick) with 2.5-cm-diam straight bore hole were placed in front of detectors to reduce exposed diameter of detector to 2.5 cm. (B) LSF for single photon counting, SPC (^{99m}Tc) system with 7-hole converging collimator and 2.5-cm-diam × 5-cm-thick NaI(Tl) detector. Line sources were in 18-cm-thick × 10-cm-wide water phantom. (Reprinted with permission from Ref. 21.)

improve the spatial resolution since the annihilation coincidence response is a function of the exposed detector diameter. It is apparent from Fig. 7-3 that the LSFs for the ACD system do not vary significantly over the full 24-cm thickness of the phantom. The full width half maximum (FWHM) resolution of the ACD response is about 40% of the exposed detector diameter (0.40 × 2.54 cm = 1.16 cm). Thus resolution can be varied by simply changing the exposed detector diameter with lead shielding. For comparison, the depth-dependent response for an SPC system with a typical converging collimator is shown in Fig. 7-3B.

If lower energy pulses are accepted by the ACD system, some deterioration in spatial resolution is observed. Phelps, et al (21) have shown that, if energies of 100 keV and above are accepted, the FWHM resolution decreases only slightly, but the full width tenth maximum (FWTM) is increased significantly because of acceptance of scattered radiation. The acceptance of scattered radiation in coincidence counting can be reduced by increasing the detector separation distance. The advantage of accepting lower energy events is the increased count rate obtained by recording 511-keV photons that reach the detector but only deposit part of their energy (by Compton interaction) in the detector.

The uniformity of depth response of SPC can be improved with suitably designed collimators (23–25) or by summing the response of two opposed detectors. Nevertheless, as pointed out by others (26–29), SPC cannot achieve the same degree of uniformity as provided by ACD.

Depth-independent sensitivity and attenuation. Annihilation coincidence detection provides depth-independent sensitivity for a plane source of positron activity in water as shown in Fig. 7-4. Constant counting sensitivity results from the fact that at different depths the solid angle to one detector increases while the solid angle to the other decreases (29). Attenuation is also constant with depth since the two 511-keV photons must always traverse the same total thickness of the object (a + b = D in Fig. 7-4) independent of their depth of origin. Therefore, absolute sensitivity can be calculated if the total thickness and the attenuation coefficient for the total material traversed are known. (Attenuation correction techniques are discussed in a later section.) This is not the case for SPC systems, such as the scintillation camera and scanner, in which both the geometric response and attenuation vary with depth (Fig. 7-3; see also Fig. 7-10). In addition, the high energy of the 511-keV photons as compared to, say, the 140-keV photons of ^{99m}Tc decreases the variations in attenuation when body substances of varying compositions and thickness are traversed.

Contrast. Typically, the most difficult objects to image in nuclear

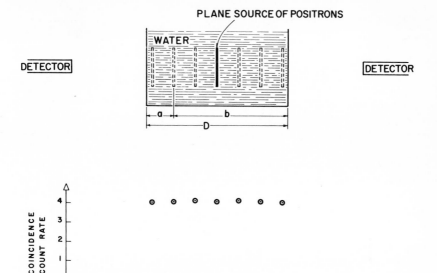

Fig. 7-4. Response of ACD system to plane source of positron-emitting radionuclide at various depths in 25-cm-thick water phantom. (Reprinted with permission from Ref. 22.)

medicine are cold spots. To illustrate the high contrast capabilities of ACD, a 2.3-cm-diam plastic rod was scanned at different depths in a water bath containing positron activity. The water bath was 18 cm long × 10 cm wide × 10 cm high. The same object was imaged using a scintillation camera with parallel-hole collimation and a scanner with a converging collimator and ^{99m}Tc in the phantom. For an ideal detector system with a constant resolution with depth of 1.1 cm and no scattered radiation accepted, the maximum decrease in count rate would be 13% at all depths. Figure 7-5 illustrates that the ACD system approximates the ideal system at all depths. The scintillation camera and scanner show exaggerated contrast at the surface but then the contrast decreases rapidly as the depth increases.

Efficiency. ACD and SPC systems employ fundamentally different types of collimation. SPC systems use absorption-type lead collimators to limit the detector field of view. Photons stopped by the collimator are lost to the image. With the electronic collimation of coincidence detection, as discussed by Burnham and Brownell (*16*), all of the photons emitted could be detected and their origins established (neglecting attenuation).

The efficiency of SPC systems increases linearly with the number of detectors used whereas with the ACD the efficiency increases with the square of the number of detectors. For example, if

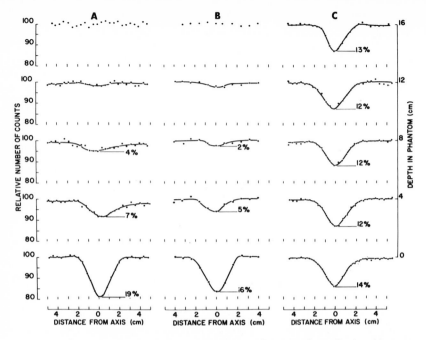

Fig. 7-5. Comparison of cold-spot scanning with 2.2-cm-diam plastic rod in water bath containing radioactive solution. (A) Scanner with absorption-type converging collimator and ^{99m}Tc (same as Fig. 7-3). Collimator-to-water bath distance was 6 cm. (B) Scintillation camera with 15,000-hole high-resolution collimator and ^{99m}Tc; phantom against face of collimator. (C) Annihilation coincidence system (same as Fig. 7-3) and ^{64}Cu. Approximately same amounts of activity and counting time were employed for each profile. (Reprinted with permission from Ref. *21*.)

SPC and ACD detector systems composed of two detectors each are increased to four detectors each, the ACD efficiency increases by a factor of 4 (Fig. 7-6). The relationship between SPC and ACD efficiency for multiple detector arrays can be generalized by the following equation:

$$R_c/R_s = K\, N^2/N = KN \qquad (2)$$

where R_c, R_s, and N are the ACD count rate, SPC count rate, and number of detector pairs, respectively. K is a proportionality constant that can be evaluated by measuring the R_c/R_s for a single pair of SPC and ACD detector systems. The value of K was determined (*21*) by placing a 20-cm-long by 1.1-cm-diam cylinder of activity between a pair of NaI(Tl) detectors with converging collimators (same collimator as employed in Fig. 7-3) and a pair of NaI(Tl) detectors connected in coincidence. Equal activities of ^{99m}Tc and ^{64}Cu were placed in the cylinder for the SPC and ACD systems, respectively. When only the photopeak was used for the ACD system the value of K was 0.12. This increased to 0.26 when the discriminator was low-

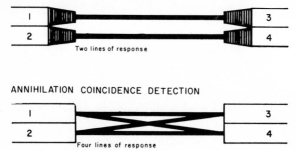

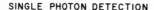

SINGLE PHOTON DETECTION

| 1 | | 3 |
| 2 | | 4 |

Two lines of response

ANNIHILATION COINCIDENCE DETECTION

| 1 | | 3 |
| 2 | | 4 |

Four lines of response

Fig. 7-6. Illustration of N and N² dependence of efficiency for SPC and ACD, respectively, for multiple detector arrays. N is number of detector pairs. (Reprinted with permission from Ref. 21.)

ered to accept all the pulses above 100 keV. Thus the single pair of SPC detectors was about four to eight times more efficient per millicurie than the ACD detector pair. Using these values of K, the ratio R_c/R_s was plotted against number of detector pairs, N (Fig. 7-7). R_c/R_s is unity with eight detector pairs for photopeak counting and with four detector pairs for counting events above 100 keV. As the number of detector pairs is further increased the ACD system rapidly increased in efficiency over the SPC system. The line K = 0.5 in Fig. 7-7 represents an upper limit, taking into account a decrease in efficiency for SPC system with more depth-independent resolution and increased coincidence detection efficiency, which could be obtained with thicker NaI(Tl) detectors than were used in this work (5 cm).

These results indicate that some conclusions from comparisons of efficiency between ACD and dual-probe scanners with SPC stated by previous investigators (*28, 30*) do not apply when a multiple coincidence scheme is employed. Further discussion and comparisons of efficiency are given by Phelps, et al (*21*).

Positron Emission Transaxial Tomograph (PETT)

A prototype transaxial tomograph employing ACD has been constructed. A schematic illustration and photograph of the system are shown in Figs. 7-8 and 7-9.

The detector system consists of 24 5.1-cm-diam × 5.1-cm-thick NaI(Tl) scintillation detectors placed in an hexagonal array (four to a side). Lead shields 2.5 cm thick with 2.5-cm-diam straight bore holes were placed in front of each detector to provide a detector resolution of about 1.1-cm FWHM (Fig. 7-3). Lead shielding was also used to exclude radiation originating outside the cross section examined. The output of each detector was connected to a separate preamplifier,

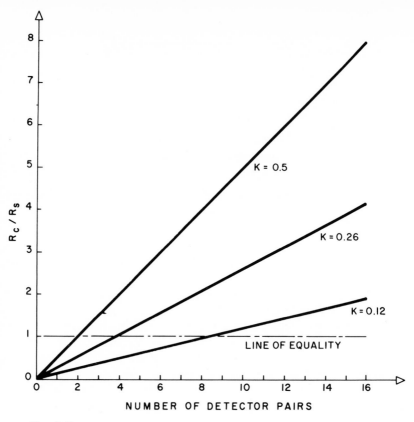

Fig. 7-7. Ratio of annihilation coincidence to single photon counting rates (R_c/R_s) vs. number of detector pairs, N. $K = (R_c/R_s)$ for single pair of detectors (see text). Line of equality indicates number of detector pairs for systems of equal efficiency.

amplifier, and single-channel analyzer. Single-channel pulse height analyzer outputs from each pair of directly opposing detectors were connected to a coincidence circuit with a resolving time of 30 nsec. With this resolving time and shielding, the highest random coincidence count rate encountered in this work was less than 5% of the true coincidence count rate. The outputs of the 12 coincidence units were routed through a parallel-channel interface to an Interdata Model 70 minicomputer.

In the prototype PETT, the object to be examined was placed at the center of the 24-detector hexagonal array on a platform that was rotated under computer control (Fig. 7-9). Coincidence data from the 12 coincident pairs of detectors were recorded every 7.5 deg through a full 360-deg rotation of the object. There was no lateral motion of the detectors, but, as a result of the offset positions of the opposing banks of detectors $(\Delta_1, \Delta_2, \Delta_3$ in Fig. 7-8), 24 data points were ob-

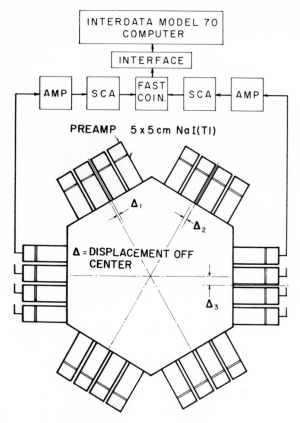

Fig. 7-8. Schematic illustration of prototype positron emission transaxial tomography system (PETT). (Reprinted with permission from Ref. 22.)

tained with a sampling resolution of 1 cm in the transverse direction at every 7.5 deg after completion of a 360-deg rotation. The data were stored and processed by the minicomputer using a Fourier-based (convolution) reconstruction algorithm (Chapter 8). The algorithm used in this work was developed by the Biomedical Computer Laboratory at Washington University School of Medicine. Data processing time of the convolution reconstruction algorithm used in this work was about 25 sec with programs written in FORTRAN.

Attenuation correction. Although the attenuation of the annihilation radiation is constant with respect to depth between two detectors in coincidence, varying thicknesses of material are interposed between each detector pair as data are collected from different angles around the object. Thus attenuation corrections must be applied. One method is to determine the physical dimensions of the object and multiply the value of each data point (coincidence count rate) by $e^{\mu x}$, where x is the thickness of the object between the coincident detector

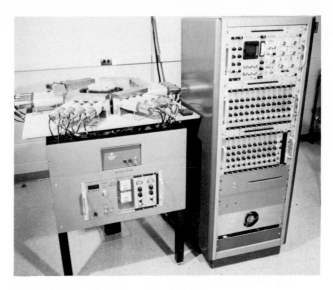

Fig. 7-9. Detector and electronics for prototype PETT. Object examined is placed on computer-controlled turntable at center of hexagon. Phantom is shown on turntable. (Reprinted with permission from Ref. 21.)

pairs, and μ is an average linear attenuation coefficient. This approach is subject to error if varying thicknesses of lung or bone are traversed although variations in μ are small for the high-energy annihilation photons. Another method consists of actually measuring the attenuation of an external 511-keV photon beam by the subject and using this information to correct the emission data before reconstruction. We have used the former method in the phantom studies; however, the latter method was used in the animal studies. A thin plastic ring containing ^{64}Cu solution was positioned around the subject and coincidence data were collected as a function of transverse and angular position. Measurements were made with and without the subject in position and the ratio of the two measurements provided an attenuation factor. Because of the well-defined, depth-independent response of annihilation coincidence detection, this attenuation correction method is accurate and simple to implement.

Phantom Studies

Spatial resolution. The spatial resolution of the prototype PETT was evaluated in terms of the resolution within the cross-sectional plane (horizontal resolution) as well as between planes (vertical resolution). Horizontal resolution was evaluated by placing three 2-mm-diam capillary tubes filled with ^{64}Cu solution in an 18-cm-diam phan-

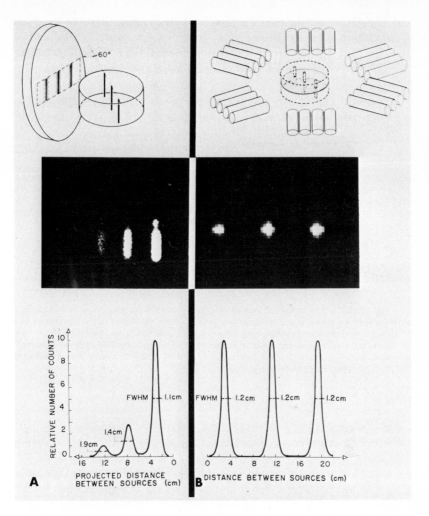

Fig. 7-10. Images and LSFs of a capillary tube and water bath phantom obtained with (A) scintillation camera (^{99m}Tc) and (B) PETT (^{64}Cu).

tom filled with water. LSFs constructed from a numerical printout of the resulting image are shown in Fig. 7-10. For comparison, the same phantom containing ^{99m}Tc was placed against the face of a Searle Radiographics camera fitted with a 15,000-hole high-resolution collimator. The phantom was oriented such that the line sources formed an angle of 60 deg with respect to the camera. The projected distance between the line sources was 4.8 cm and they were 2, 9, and 16 cm from the face of the camera. Numerical data collected by a digital computer interfaced to the camera were used to construct the LSFs shown in Fig. 7-10. This illustrates the depth-independent resolution and sensitivity of the PETT in the horizontal plane and the decrease in resolution and sensitivity with depth of the scintillation camera. The FWHM resolution of the reconstructed PETT image was only slightly less than that of a single pair of coincident detectors (Fig. 7-3).

Vertical resolution was evaluated with a phantom having two separate compartments in the vertical direction (Fig. 7-11). The lower

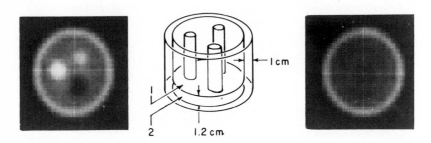

Fig. 7-11. Evaluation of vertical resolution of PETT scanner. (Center) Drawing of plastic phantom. (Left) Image obtained at level 1, which contained relative activities 3, 1, 5, 3, and 0 in 1-cm-diam outside ring, 14-cm-diam inside container, two 2-cm-diam "hot" cylinders and one 3-cm-diam "cold" cylinder. (Right) Image obtained at level 2, containing outside ring and inside container only. A total of 300,000 counts was acquired for each image. (Reprinted with permission from Ref. 21.)

compartment was 1.2-cm thick and contained a ring of activity surrounding a cylinder of uniformly less activity. The upper section contained the same ring and cylinder of activity as well as two 2-cm-diam hot sections and one 3-cm-diam cold section. Data collected with the PETT from the upper and lower sections of the phantom were reconstructed and the resulting images are shown in Fig. 7-11. The image from the lower section does not show any of the structure of the upper section, which was only 6 mm from the center of the lower section. Thus, the PETT displayed excellent vertical resolution.

Quantitative and cold spot images. The ability of the PETT to yield quantitative images was tested with a 14-cm-diam phantom filled with positron-emitting radioactivity. Two 3-cm-diam tubes inside the phantom contained activity concentrations 0 and 4 relative to the surrounding solution. The reconstructed relative activity levels for the phantom and two cylinders were 1 ± 0.1, 0 ± 0.1, and 4 ± 0.1, which were in excellent agreement with the actual relative activities in the phantom (21). The 3-cm-diam objects were employed to demonstrate the quantitative aspect of the reconstruction since the sampling resolution (~ 1 cm) must be at least two times finer than the object size for quantitative reconstruction in accordance with the sampling theorem (*31*) as discussed in Chapter 8.

To further evaluate the accuracy of cold spot reconstruction with the PETT, another 14-cm-diam phantom was filled with ^{64}Cu, and voids (tubes filled with water) of 1-, 2-, 3-, and 3.5-cm diam were placed in the phantom. All the voids were visible in the reconstructed image and the reconstruction of activities was zero, except for the 1-cm void. Thus, the 1-cm detector resolution employed in this study did not recover the quantitative value for a 1-cm-diam object, as predicted by the sampling theorem.

Comparison of the PETT and scintillation camera. Comparative images of a 6-cm-thick phantom obtained with a scintillation camera and with the PETT are shown in Fig. 7-12 for equal activities of

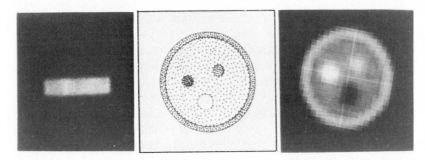

Fig. 7-12. Comparison of images obtained on phantom with Anger camera (^{99m}Tc) and PETT scanner (^{64}Cu). (Center) Cross section of phantom, comprised of 1-cm-diam outside ring, 14-cm-diam inside, two 2-cm-diam "hot" cylinders, and one 3-cm-diam "cold" cylinder. (Left) Anger camera image, with phantom against face of 15,000-hole high-resolution collimator. (Right) PETT scanner image. (Reprinted with permission from Ref. 22.)

^{99m}Tc and ^{64}Cu, respectively. Both images contain 300,000 counts, but the camera collection time for the 6-cm-thick slice was 16 min versus 12 min for a 1-cm-thick slice with the PETT. Superior definition of the PETT for both hot and cold lesions is apparent.

Animal Studies

Several studies were carried out in dogs to assess the capabilities of the PETT for visualization of intravenously administered positron-emitting radiopharmaceuticals and to demonstrate the importance of attenuation corrections.

An experiment was carried out in the following sequence: The dog was intravenously injected with 10 mCi of $H_2^{15}O$ (^{15}O, half-life = 2 min). Three minutes was allowed for equilibration with the rapidly equilibrating water compartments, and then a 4.8-min image was recorded from a 1-cm-thick cross section at the level of the sixth thoracic vertebra. Twelve millicuries of $^{13}NH_3$(^{13}N, half-life = 10 min) was injected intravenously and 8 min was allowed for the clearance of the ammonia from the blood and equilibration in soft tissues. Another image was recorded with a data collection period of 12 min. The dog was then allowed to breathe ^{11}CO (^{11}C, half-life = 20.4 min) for about 1 min to label the blood with approximately 8 mCi of ^{11}CO-hemoglobin. Five minutes was allowed for equilibration in the blood pool before a 24-min data collection period. (The production of the positron-labeled compounds is described in Chapter 3.)

A sketch showing anatomical structure is at the upper left-hand corner of Fig. 7-13. These structures were identified by anteroposterior and lateral x-ray films and at autopsy. The reconstructed images at the top of Fig. 7-13 were corrected for attenuation by the transmission method described earlier. Transmission data were also processed in the reconstruction algorithm and the resulting image is also shown in Fig. 7-13. The image taken with $H_2^{15}O$ shows the distribution of equilibrated water in soft tissue. The equilibration of bone water is slow, accounting for the void in the image at the position of the vertebral column. The lungs also show a relatively low concentration of $H_2^{15}O$. The $^{13}NH_3$ is preferentially taken up in the myocardium as reported by others (32, 33). Image contrast between the myocardium and the surrounding soft tissue is about 8 to 1. The ^{11}CO-hemoglobin image demonstrates the blood distribution in the chambers of the heart and large blood vessels and the general blood distribution in surrounding tissues.

The $H_2^{15}O$, $^{13}NH_3$, and ^{11}CO images in the lower portion of Fig. 7-13 were not corrected for attenuation. Note that the outer boundaries in these images are incorrect and that prominent structures are distorted. The lungs in the $H_2^{15}O$ image have moved and almost disappeared in the image.

The same sequence of injections and data collections was carried out on a second dog at the level of the eleventh thoracic vertebra (Fig. 7-14). The $^{13}NH_3$ image shows the concentration of ammonia in the liver that is probably a result of its incorporation into the urea cycle. The ^{11}CO-hemoglobin image shows the blood distribution in the liver, spleen, and large blood vessels. The voids are the small intestine and stomach. The $H_2^{15}O$ image shows the equilibrated water in soft tissue.

The images in Figs. 7-13 and 7-14 were generated without any correction for cardiac or respiratory motion.

PETT III

The prototype PETT utilized only the coincidences between directly opposing pairs of detectors (total of 12 coincident pairs).

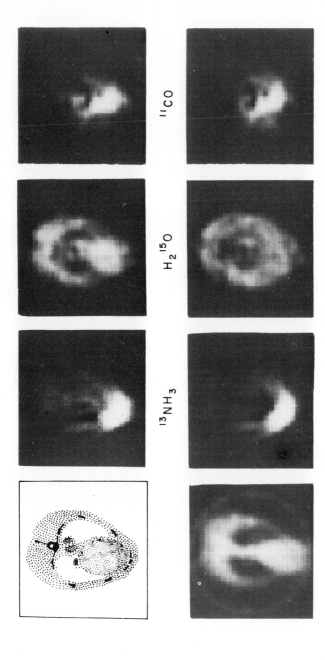

Fig. 7-13. Reconstructed images for 1-cm-thick cross section of dog at level of sixth thoracic vertebra after intravenous injection of $H_2^{15}O$, $^{13}NH_3$, and ^{11}CO. Images contained 63,000, 230,000, and 350,000 counts, respectively. Sketch of anatomic structure is shown at upper left and reconstructed transmission image is shown at lower left. Top row images were corrected for attenuation based on transmission scan data; bottom row images were not. (Reprinted with permission from Ref. 21.)

However, a more efficient design employs multiple coincidences between all the detectors on opposing sides of the hexagon. The PETT III employs this type of coincidence logic (Fig. 7-15) with a total of 48 5-cm-diam × 7.5-cm-thick NaI(Tl) detectors. This yields a total of 192 coincident pairs of detectors. A photograph of PETT III is shown in Fig. 7-16. The center hole through which the patient is passed is 50 cm diam and will accommodate the human head or torso. Cross-sectional and vertical (slice thickness) resolution can be varied from 5 mm to 2 cm simply by changing a 2.5-cm-thick lead collimator in front of the detectors. The patient remains stationary on the table and the detector gantry rotates in 3-deg increments through an angle of 60 deg. The detectors scan through a linear motion of 5 cm at each angle. All scanning motions, data collection, processing, and display are under control of an on-line minicomputer.

The increased efficiency of the PETT III over the prototype PETT should allow the cross-sectional tomographic examination to be carried out in 1–2 min/slice with 1-cm resolution following the intravenous injection of approximately 10 mCi of a positron-labeled radiopharmaceutical.

The results of some preliminary studies carried out on the PETT III are shown in Fig. 7-17. Figure 7-17A shows a reconstructed image obtained on a normal human subject 1 cm above the level of the orbital meatal line after inhalation of 20 mCi of ^{11}CO to produce ^{11}C-labeled hemoglobin. The image was obtained 3 min after inhalation to allow for equilibration of the blood tracer. A total of 1.5 million counts was recorded in a 2-min imaging time. Prominent structures seen in the image are the superior sagittal sinus, right and left lateral sinuses, and internal carotid arteries. The general blood distribution in cerebral and extracerebral tissues is also seen. Figure 7-17B shows a reconstructed image obtained on the same subject at a level 4 cm above the orbital meatal line, 20 min after intravenous injection of 1 mCi of ^{11}C-labeled glucose. A total of 350,000 counts was recorded in 10 min for this image. Figure 7-17C is a cerebral perfusion image with $^{13}NH_3$ at the same level as the ^{11}C-glucose image. Fifteen millicuries was injected intravenously and about 1,000,000 counts were recorded in 4 min. Note the high glucose uptake and high perfusion in the region of the cortex. The ratio of $^{13}NH_3$ in cortex to subcortical white matter is 2.9, in excellent agreement with the ratio of 3 for normal flows in these regions.

Future Potential for CRTT Scanning

As discussed in Chapter 8, the dramatic improvement in radiographic imaging demonstrated by the EMI scanner resulted not only from the transaxial reconstruction algorithm but also from the high

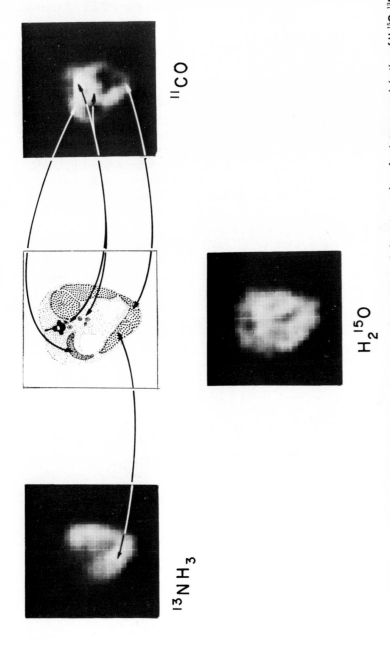

^{11}CO

$H_2^{15}O$

$^{13}NH_3$

Fig. 7-14. Reconstructed images for 1-cm-thick cross section of dog at level of eleventh thoracic vertebra after intravenous injection of $H_2^{15}O$, $^{13}NH_3$, and ^{11}CO. Images contained 55,000, 205,000, and 232,000 counts, respectively. Sketch of anatomic structure is shown at center (see text). (Reprinted with permission from Ref. 22.)

contrast narrow-beam scanning technique and the quantitative detection system. The same improvements are possible in radionuclide imaging with the ACD techniques employed in the PETT. Removal of the superpositioning of information will also provide significant improvement in the quality of nuclear medicine images.

The quantitative imaging capability of the PETT scanner provides a means for carrying out accurate determinations of physiological variables with appropriate radiopharmaceuticals (Chapters 3 and 5). In addition, the quantitative capabilities of the system result in an image contrast equal to the object contrast provided the object size is larger than about twice the system resolution.

The fact that the PETT is limited to positron-emitting radionuclides might appear to be a limiting factor in its application in clinical nuclear medicine. However, there are a number of positron-emitting radionuclides with favorable physical and chemical properties. A commercial generator system is available for ^{68}Ga (half-life = 1.1 hr) from the long-lived parent ^{68}Ge (half-life = 272 days). Gallium-68 could be used in a number of existing procedures such as ^{68}Ga-DTPA or ^{68}Ga-EDTA for brain and kidney, ^{68}Ga(OH)$_3$ particles, or ^{68}Ga-macroaggregated albumin for lung, liver, and spleen studies. It should also be possible to bind ^{68}Ga to the pyro- or polyphosphates for bone or myocardial scanning agents. A number of positron-emitting radionuclides, such as ^{11}C, ^{13}N, ^{15}O, and ^{18}F, currently employed in

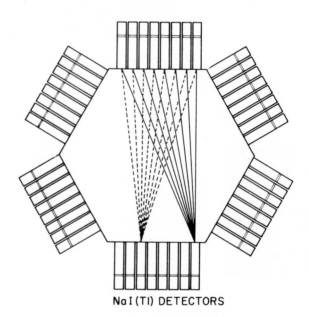

NaI(Tl) DETECTORS

Fig. 7-15. Multiple coincidence logic of PETT III. (Reprinted with permission from Ref. 21.)

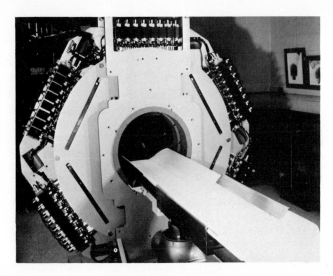

Fig. 7-16. PETT III tomographic scanner for head and whole-body studies of human subjects.

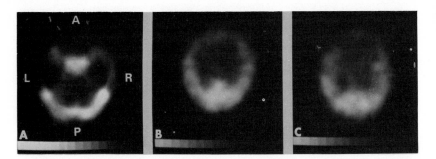

Fig. 7-17. Cross-sectional images of brain of normal human subject obtained with PETT III. (A) Image obtained at level 1 cm above orbital meatal line 3 min after inhalation of ^{11}CO to produce ^{11}C-labeled hemoglobin. (B) Image obtained at level 4 cm above orbital meatal line 20 min after injection of ^{11}C-labeled glucose. (C) Cerebral perfusion image with ^{13}NH$_3$. Same level as (B).

physiological studies in conjunction with the quantitative feature of the PETT offer the potential of assessing the metabolic status of an organ (or regions of an organ). In general the dedication of this system to positron-emitting radionuclides may be less restrictive than the low photon energy requirement imposed by the scintillation camera and scanner and the limitations imposed by the chemical properties of technetium.

Acknowledgments

We thank J.R. Cox and D. Snyder for the development of the algorithm and discussions, H. Huang for many helpful discussions of the algorithm, J. Hood and J. Hecht for technical assistance, C. Coble for programming, and E. Coleman and B. Siegel for discussions and help in animal preparations. This work was partially supported by NIH Grants 5-PO1-HL13 851 and 1-RO1-HL15423 and by NIH fellowship 1F03 GM 55196-01.

References

1. KUHL DE, EDWARDS RQ: Image separation radioisotope scanning. *Radiology* 80: 653–662, 1963

2. KUHL DE, EDWARDS RQ: Reorganizing data from transverse section scans using digital processing. *Radiology* 91: 975–983, 1968

3. KUHL DE, EDWARDS RQ: The Mark III scanner. A compact device for multiview and section scanning of the brain. *Radiology* 96: 563–570, 1970

4. KUHL DE, EDWARDS RQ, RICCI AR, et al: Quantitative section scanning using orthogonal tangent correction. *J Nucl Med* 14: 196–200, 1973

5. TODD-POKROPEK AE: Tomography and the reconstruction of images from their projections. In *Proceedings of the Third International Conference on Data Handling and Image Processing in Scintigraphy,* Metz C, ed, 1973

6. TODD-POKROPEK AE: The formation and display of section scans. In *Proceedings of Symposium of American Congress of Radiology*, 1971, Amsterdam, Excerpta Medica, 1972, p 545

7. BOWLEY AR, TAYLOR CG, CAUSER DA, et al: A radioisotope scanner for rectilinear, arc, transverse section and longitudinal section scanning. (ASS-The Aberdeen Section Scanner.) *Br J Radiol* 46: 262–271, 1973

8. MYERS MJ, KEYES WI, MALLARD JR: An analysis of tomographic scanning systems. In *Medical Radioisotope Scintigraphy,* vol 2, Vienna, IAEA, 1972, pp 331–345

9. TANAKA E: Multi-crystal section imaging device and its data processing. In *Proceedings of the Thirteenth Congress in Radiology,* Amsterdam, Excerpta Medica, 1973, p 81

10. TANAKA E, SHIMIZU T, IINUMA T, et al: Digital simulation of section image resconstruction. National Institute of Radiological Science, Tokyo, Report NIRS-12, 1973, pp 3–4

11. BUDINGER TF, GULLBERG GT: Three-dimensional reconstruction in nuclear medicine by iterative least-squares and Fourier transform techniques. *IEEE Trans Nucl Sci* NS-21: 2–20, 1974

12. BUDINGER TF, GULLBERG GT: Three-dimensional reconstruction of isotope distributions. *Phys Med Biol* 19: 387–389, 1974

13. OPPENHEIM BE, HARPER PV: Iterative three-dimensional reconstruction: a search for a better algorithm. *J Nucl Med* 15: 520, 1974

14. KEYES JW, KAY DB, SIMON W: Digital reconstruction of three-dimensional radionuclide images. *J Nucl Med* 14: 628–629, 1973

15. BROWNELL GL, BURNHAM CA, WILENSKY S, et al: New developments in positron scintigraphy and the application of cyclotron-produced positron emitters. In *Medical Radioisotope Scintigraphy,* vol 1, Vienna, IAEA, 1968, pp 163–176

16. BURNHAM CA, BROWNELL GL: A multicrystal positron camera. *IEEE Med Sci* NS19 3: 201–205, 1973

17. CHESLER DA: Three-dimensional activity distribution from multiple positron scintigraphs. *J Nucl Med* 12: 347–348, 1971

18. CHESLER DA: Positron tomography and three-dimensional reconstruction techniques. In *Tomographic Imaging in Nuclear Medicine*, Freedman GS, ed, New York, Society of Nuclear Medicine, 1973, pp 176–183

19. ROBERTSON JS, MARR RB, ROSENBAUM M, et al: Thirty-two crystal positron transverse section detector. In *Tomographic Imaging in Nuclear Medicine*, Freedman GS, ed, New York, Society of Nuclear Medicine, 1973, pp 142–153

20. CORMACK AM: Reconstruction of densities from their projections, with applications in radiological physics. *Phys Med Biol* 18: 195–207, 1973

21. PHELPS ME, HOFFMAN EJ, MULLANI N, et al: Application of annihilation coincidence detection to transaxial reconstruction tomography. *J Nucl Med* 16: 210–224, 1975

22. TER-POGOSSIAN MM, PHELPS ME, HOFFMAN EJ, et al: A positron emission transaxial tomography for nuclear medicine imaging. *Radiology* 114: 89–98, 1975

23. BECK, RN: Collimation of gamma rays. In *Fundamental Problems in Scanning*, Gottschalk A, Beck RN, eds, Springfield, Ill, Charles C Thomas, 1968, pp 71–92

24. GENNA S, FARMELANT MH, BURROWS BA: Improved scintiscan resolution without sensitivity loss: "Constant resolution" collimator. In *Medical Radioisotope Scintigraphy*, vol 1, Vienna, IAEA, 1968, pp 561–574

25. CLARKE LP, LAUGHLIN JS, MAYER K: Quantitative organ-uptake measurement. *Radiology* 102: 375–382, 1972

26. WRENN R, GOOD ML, HANDLER P: The use of positron-emitting radioisotopes for the localization of brain tumors. *Science* 113: 525, 1951

27. BROWNELL GL, SWEET WH: Localization of brain tumors with positron emitters. *Nucleonics* 11: 40–45, 1953

28. MATTHEWS CME: Comparison of coincidence counting and focusing collimators with various isotopes in brain tumor detection. *Br J Radiol* 37: 531, 1964

29. BROWNELL GL: Theory of radioisotope scanning. *Int J Appl Radiat Isot* 3: 181–192, 1958

30. BECK RN: A theoretical evaluation of brain scanning systems. *J Nucl Med* 2: 314–324, 1961

31. HANCOCK JC: *An Introduction to the Principles of Communication Theory*, New York, McGraw-Hill, 1951, p 18

32. HARPER PV, LATHROP KA, KRIZEK H, et al: Clinical feasibility of myocardial imaging with $^{13}NH_3$. *J Nucl Med* 13: 278–281, 1972

33. MONAHAN WG, TILBURY RS, LAUGHLIN JS: Uptake of ^{13}N-labeled ammonia. *J Nucl Med* 13: 274–277, 1972

Chapter 8

Computerized Transaxial Transmission Reconstruction Tomography

Michael E. Phelps, Edward J. Hoffman,
Mokhtar Gado, and Michel M. Ter-Pogossian

Imaging in diagnostic radiology has generally employed methods in which a two-dimensional projection is taken of a three-dimensional body. Many improvements have been made in imaging devices such as increasing their resolution, linearity, uniformity, and contrast, and shortening the examination time. However, most of these improvements have been directed toward the two-dimensional aspect of the imaging device, with the result that the third dimension, depth, occurs as a superposition of information in the image. The conventional method of assessing the depth of structures in the body is to record multiple images from different orthogonal views (e.g., anteroposterior and lateral). It is then left to the viewer to visually sort out the three-dimensional aspect of the object. The situation is further complicated by the limitations of imaging systems to display information accurately if a large range or latitude of information is present from the third dimension of depth.

The minimization or removal of the superposition of information with depth has been the purpose of a number of tomographic techniques over the past 50 years, which were aimed at producing an image of a section of the body at a given depth. Until recently, tomographic images in radiology were produced by using variations of "focal plane" tomography first described by Bocage in 1921. In this type of tomography the x-ray tube and film are held on a rigid support and moved synchronously in opposite directions with the fulcrum of the motion at the plane of interest (focal plane). Structures in the focal plane are recorded in focus throughout the motion whereas structures in planes above and below are blurred by the motion (*1*). Many different types of coupled motion of x-ray tube and film have been employed, including linear, circular, elliptical, and hypocycloidal (*2, 3*). This type of tomography has also been utilized for radionuclide imaging (*4*).

Even though focal plane tomography has been successful, there are four major factors that limit its usefulness in diagnostic radiology: (A) The degree of blurring or defocusing is progressive, increasing with distance away from the focal plane. This creates a preference for the focal plane but not a distinct defocusing cutoff. (B) The recorded image contains the superposition of the focal plane structure and the blurred structures from planes above and below, limiting the perception of low-contrast objects in the focal plane. (C) The perception of low-contrast objects is further limited by the recording of scattered radiation and x-ray film-screen limitations (e.g., nonuniformities, film base-plus-fog density, nonlinearity). (D) Artifactual images of non-focal plane structures may be produced because of tube-film motion.

The type of tomography to be discussed here is called computerized transaxial transmission reconstruction tomography (CTT). The term transaxial means that the tomographic plane or section is perpendicular to the long axis of the body. In this type of tomography a narrow collimated beam of x-rays from an x-ray tube is scanned across the plane or cross section of interest in a transverse fashion at various discrete angles, θ (Fig. 8-1). The transverse scans are repeated through a full 180 deg. The transmitted x-ray intensity is measured by a NaI(Tl) scintillation detector and reflects the attenuation of the x-ray beam in the material traversed. The data collected in this manner are processed by a mathematical algorithm with a computer to generate a cross-sectional display related to the attenuation coefficients in the examined slice.

Before describing this technique in detail, it should be pointed out that a number of the limitations of focal plane tomography are removed in transaxial reconstruction tomography as follows: (A) The x-ray beam is passed through the cross section of interest only, and thus the image does not contain the superposition of information from planes above or below. (B) The contrast limitation imposed on focal plane tomography by the inclusion of scattered radiation and the limitations of x-ray film-screen combinations are removed by the use of a narrow x-ray beam scanning technique ("good scatter geometry") and a quantitative radiation detector.

Some of the limitations of transaxial tomography will also be discussed later in the chapter.

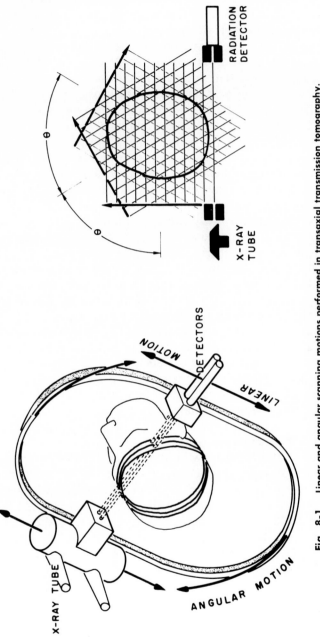

RADIATION DETECTOR

X-RAY TUBE

DETECTORS

LINEAR MOTION

X-RAY TUBE

ANGULAR MOTION

Fig. 8-1. Linear and angular scanning motions performed in transaxial transmission tomography.

EMI Scanner*

The EMI scanner (5, 6) will be used to illustrate the basic principles of CTT scanning. The EMI scanner employs a collimated x-ray tube and two collimated NaI(Tl) detectors rigidly mounted on a frame or gantry (Fig. 8-1). The x-ray tube is typically operated at 120–140 kVp and at corresponding currents of 35–25 mA. The NaI(Tl) detectors record the transmitted x-ray intensity from the two narrow collimated beams of x-rays passing through the cross section of the head. The x-ray beam is collimated to approximately 3 mm wide by 8 or 13 mm high (thickness of the slice), and two contiguous slices are examined simultaneously. A linear scan is performed, and 240 discrete readings are taken by each of the two NaI(Tl) detectors (approximately one reading per millimeter). At the end of the scan the gantry is rotated 1 deg and another linear scan is performed. This sequence continues through 180 deg, resulting in a total of 43,200 (180 × 240) readings of transmitted x-ray intensity for each detector.† A third NaI(Tl) detector is employed as a reference to detect variations in the output of the x-ray tube (Fig. 8-2).

Because of the high intensity of the recorded x-ray beam ($\sim 2 \times 10^7$ cps), the NaI(Tl) detectors cannot count pulses and are instead operated in a direct current (dc) integration mode. The dc output signals from the detectors are digitized with an analog-to-digital converter (ADC). The computer processes the digitized data with an appropriate algorithm to determine the distribution of attenuation coefficients in the examined cross sections of the brain. These data are converted to analog form with a digital-to-analog converter (DAC) for display on a cathode-ray tube for viewing and photographing. Numerical values related to the attenuation coefficients can also be printed out by a line printer.

In the EMI scanner the patient's head is held with a rubber cap in a water box so that the narrow beam of x-rays always passes through a fixed length of water or water plus the head. The reference detector is placed behind an aluminum absorber that reduces the reference beam intensity to a value equal to the intensity transmitted through the water box. Thus the reference beam not only normalizes for x-ray tube variations but also allows the calculation of attenuation coefficients relative to the value for water. A water box is not used in some CTT scanners [e.g., ACTA (7) and Ohio-Nuclear]. Information on the amount by which the reference beam is attenuated in these systems is not generally available at this time. Further discussion of

---

* In this book all references to the "EMI Scanner" pertain to the EMI brain-scanning device.

† The first version of EMI scanner took 160 discrete readings during each linear scan at 1-deg angles, yielding 28,800 (180 × 160) readings for each slice.

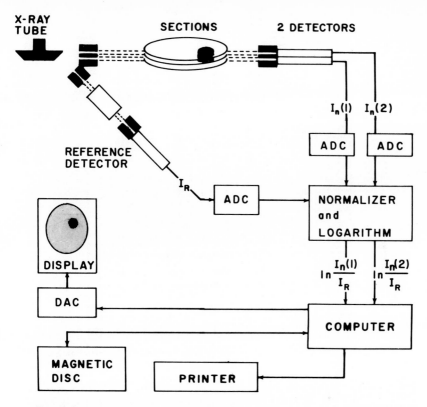

Fig. 8-2. Schematic arrangement of radiation detectors, electronics, and computer system employed in the EMI scanner. $I_n(1)$, $I_n(2)$ are current outputs of two radiation detectors recording transmitted x-ray intensity from two slices. I_R is current output from reference detector. ADC and DAC are analog-to-digital and digital-to-analog converters, respectively.

the water box is given in later sections of this chapter. More complete descriptions of the operational characteristics of the EMI and ACTA scanners are given by Hounsfield (5, 6) and Ledley, et al (7), respectively.

Reconstruction Algorithms

The basic approach in CTT scanning is to use the x-ray intensities transmitted at different angles through the brain to determine the attenuation coefficients for each of the cells in a matrix representation of the cross section examined (Fig. 8-3). The attenuation coefficient, μ, for the passage of x-rays through matter can be determined from:

$$I_n/I_o = e^{-\mu x} \tag{1}$$

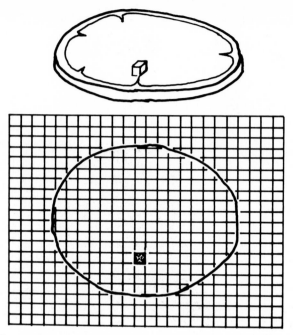

Fig. 8-3. Grid or matrix representation of tomographic cross section of brain.

where I_o and I_n are incident and x-ray intensities and x is the total thickness of the material traversed. If the pathlength of the x-ray beam is then broken up into small cells of equal thicknesses, Δx, Eq. 1 can be written as:

$$I_n/I_o = e^{-\sum_i^{} \mu_i \Delta x} \tag{2}$$

where μ_i are the attenuation coefficients for individual cells.

In the EMI scanner an aluminum absorber reduces the x-ray intensity at the reference detector to a value, I_R, equal to that recorded by the other two detectors when only water is traversed (Fig. 8-2). Thus, the measured intensities, I_n and I_R, are related as:

$$(I_n/I_o)/(I_R/I_o) = e^{-\sum_i^{} \mu_i \Delta x}/e^{-\mu_w x}. \tag{3}$$

Since $e^{-\mu_w x}$ can be written as $e^{-\sum_i^{} \mu_w \Delta x}$, Eq. 3 reduces to:

$$I_n/I_R = e^{-\sum_i^{}(\mu_i - \mu_w)\Delta x}. \tag{4}$$

Taking the natural logarithm yields:

$$\ln(I_n/I_R) = -\sum_i (\mu_i - \mu_w) \Delta x. \tag{5}$$

Thus, in the EMI scanner the difference between the tissue attenuation coefficient (μ_i) and the value for water (μ_w) is calculated and not the absolute value for the tissue.

In the EMI scanner $\ln(I_n/I_R)$ is calculated in a unit separate from the computer (Fig. 8-2) for each reading taken during a linear scan. Data taken at different linear and angular positions are then used to compute the attenuation coefficients for each of the cells in the matrix or grid.

Two basic assumptions of Eqs. 1–5 are that the source is monoenergetic (or behaves as though it were) and that the x-ray interactions in the material traversed are absorption interactions (no variations in the amount of accepted scattered radiation). The assumptions are examined in detail in later sections.

Algebraic algorithms. The general problem of reconstruction algorithms has been reviewed by Gordon and Herman (8). The first objective of the algorithm is to reduce the three-dimensional problem to a set of one-dimensional calculations. This is accomplished by first assuming that the slice has no thickness and is thus a two-dimensional plane. Then each transverse scan is represented as a series of one-dimensional equations, in which each detector reading represents the attenuation along a line across the plane.

A simple example of an algebraic reconstruction is shown in Fig. 8-4 for a 2×2 grid with four unknowns, x_1 to x_4. If one views the object from the four positions shown to obtain readings y_1 to y_4, the following equations can be written:

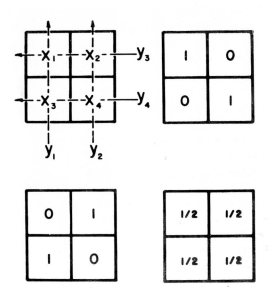

Fig. 8-4. Simple example of nonunique reconstruction solutions obtained when data are taken only at orthogonal positions. x_1 to x_4 are cell contents and y_1 to y_4 are readings. Three examples shown for cell contents all give same readings, y_1 to $y_4 = 1$.

$$y_1 = x_1 + x_3$$
$$y_2 = x_2 + x_4$$
$$y_3 = x_1 + x_2$$
$$y_4 = x_3 + x_4. \tag{6}$$

These are four equations in four unknowns, x_1 to x_4. However, the solution of this set of equations yields only the requirement that:

$$x_1 - x_2 = x_3 - x_4 \tag{7}$$

which does not give a unique solution for the values of x_1 to x_4. For example, the three distributions shown in Fig. 8-4 could all be obtained from the same set of equations. Thus, the criteria of n equations for n unknowns is not enough. They must be n *independent* equations. The ambiguity in Fig. 8-4 could be removed by taking measurements along diagonal positions. In general it is important that enough data be collected to obtain unique solutions for all the unknowns, such that an unambiguous result is obtained.

There are, of course, many more than four equations in a CTT problem. One approach for solving a large set of equations is by matrix inversion. However, matrix inversion of a CTT problem (e.g., 160×160 attenuation coefficient array) would require a computer large enough to handle $(160 \times 160)^2 = 6.6 \times 10^8$ numbers. Therefore, other algebraic calculation schemes have been developed to minimize computation requirements.

A starting point for these methods is called linear superposition of back projections (LSBP), which is illustrated in Fig. 8-5 for a cross section of a three-dimensional object scanned in transaxial fashion. For simplicity, it is assumed that detector readings are zero everywhere except at the dark cyclinder. Each detector reading is spread across the image (e.g., on a film or cathode-ray tube display) at the position where it was taken (back projection). This is repeated at different angles with the back projection from each angle simply added to the image (linear superposition). The resulting images from three and six (many) angular scans are shown at the bottom of Fig. 8-5. The position of the cylinder is apparent because there is reinforcement of back projections from different angles. This is the original approach employed by Kuhl and Edwards (9). However, this technique is not satisfactory because there are nonzero values in the image, where actual values in the examined cross section are zero. This is a type of noise that results in a blurring or defocusing of the image, similar to the situation in focal plane tomography. Corrective techniques can be applied to remove this "defocusing" effect as described in the discussion of Fourier techniques to come.

Another algebraic approach is represented by the orthogonal tangent correction technique of Kuhl and Edwards (10) and by the more sophisticated iterative approaches of Hounsfield (6), Gordon, et

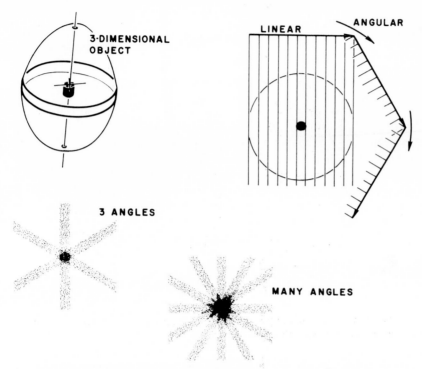

Fig. 8-5. Example of linear superposition of back-projected data (LSBP) taken in transaxial tomography. Attenuation reading is assumed to be zero except when dark cylinder is encountered. Even with many angles object is blurred, and inaccurate (nonzero) values are reconstructed outside the object image.

al (*11*), Gilbert (*12*), and Meyers (*13*). The specific techniques of these authors will not be discussed, but a generalized example of the iterative approach will be given to illustrate the basic principles. The general technique is known as the algebraic reconstruction technique (ART).

Consider the 6×6 grid (36-grid elements) shown in Fig. 8-6 and the following definitions:

1. b_{ij} is an attenuation value for the contents of cell (i, j). This may be an assumed value (initial starting point) or a value obtained by calculation after one or more iterations.
2. $A_{ij\theta}$ is the total attenuation recorded for a reading at angle θ passing through cell (i, j).
3. $f_{ij\theta}$ is the fraction of cell (i, j) in the beam where the reading $A_{ij\theta}$ is recorded.
4. $N_{ij\theta}$ is the total number of cells viewed by the detector where the reading is $A_{ij\theta}$ ($N_{ij\theta} = \Sigma f_{ij\theta}$).

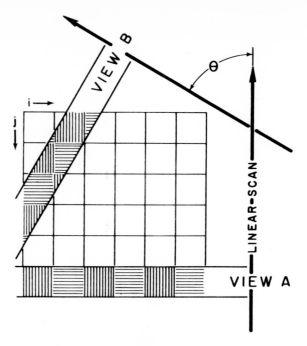

Fig. 8-6. A 6 × 6 grid (36 grid elements) illustrating general reconstruction approach employed in algebraic iterative algorithms.

5. $B_{ij\theta} = \Sigma b_{hk} f_{hk\theta}$ is a calculated sum of attenuation values over all cells (h, k) in the beam where the reading $A_{ij\theta}$ is recorded, modified by their fractional area in the beam, $f_{hk\theta}$.

Two calculations are then performed for each value of $A_{ij\theta}$ recorded in a scan.

Step 1: Calculate $(A_{ij\theta} - B_{ij\theta})/N_{ij\theta}$.
Step 2: Add the value calculated in step 1 multiplied by the factor $f_{ij\theta}$ to the content of each cell in the beam where the reading $A_{ij\theta}$ was recorded.

For example, consider the grid shown in Fig. 8-6. Assume that the values for all the grid elements are initially set equal to 2. Suppose the first detector reading, along view A, is 42. For this row, $f_{ij\theta} = 1$ for all of the elements, since the full area of each element is viewed. Therefore, the calculations are as follows:

Step 1: $(42 - 12)/6 = 5$.
Step 2: The value 5 is added to the previously existing value, 2, for all the elements in the first column.

These calculations are repeated for each detector reading across the first scan, and then repeated again for all of the other linear scans recorded at other viewing angles around the grid. A complete set of calculations including data from all viewing angles is called an iteration. The iteration process is repeated several times or until some criteria in the algorithm is satisfied, such as minimal change from one iteration to the next. In CTT scanning, $A_{ij\theta}$ corresponds to a measured value of $\ln(I_n/I_R)$ and b_{ij} corresponds to a number proportional to the attenuation coefficient for the cell.

Proper application of this technique has been shown to eliminate the defocusing obtained with simple back projections (11–13). It is similar to the technique used in early versions of the EMI scanner.

Another algebraic approach, developed by Gilbert (12), is referred to as SIRT (simultaneous iterative reconstruction technique). SIRT differs from ART in that the value for the content of a cell is calculated by simultaneously including data from all those views that have crossed the grid element in question. Thus, a value is calculated for a single grid element in an iterative fashion, then the next grid element, and so on, until all elements have been evaluated.

Fourier-based algorithms. Fourier-based reconstruction algorithms offer a more direct approach to the solution of the CTT reconstruction problem (14, 15). These techniques include the use of Fourier series, Fourier transforms, convolutions, or, equivalently, filtering of scan profiles before back-projection. They have been used for medical applications by a number of authors (16–20) and are also used in newer versions of commercial CTT systems. The basic principles of Fourier techniques will be illustrated using the linear superposition of filtered back-projections (LSFBP) technique.

Linear scans taken at different angles yield attenuation profiles of the examined cross section. Referring to Fig. 8-7 assume that the attenuation readings are zero except when the small object in the center is encountered. Thus, each linear scan yields an attenuation profile with a single positive response. Simple back-projection of these profiles would result in a blurred image similar to that shown in Fig. 8-5. This effect results from the fact that the high-frequency components of the cross-sectional image are attenuated by a factor proportional to their spatial frequency. To compensate for this, each scan profile is filtered by a function that enhances different frequency components by a factor proportional to their spatial frequency (Fig. 8-7B). The filtered scan profile is then projected back across the cross-sectional plane. When this process is repeated for four scan angles the result shown in Fig. 8-7C is obtained. Four scan angles are insufficient to remove all the defocusing (only the noise close to the object is reduced). However, the situation is progressively improved as the number of angles is increased. When data from a sufficient

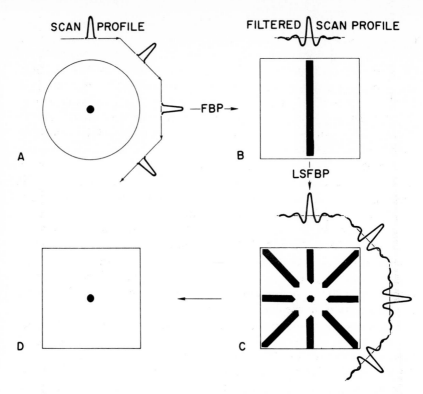

Fig. 8-7. Example of Fourier-based reconstruction technique, linear superposition of filtered back-projections (LSFBP). Detector readings are zero except when small object at center is encountered. (A) Object and scan profiles. (B) Single filtered scan profile projected back across cross-sectional plane. Note positive and negative components of filtered profile. (C) Four filtered scan profiles projected back across plane and added together (superposition). (D) Image produced when sufficient angles are employed to remove defocusing.

number of angles are used (see the discussion on sampling that follows) in the linear superposition of filtered back projections (LSFBP), the correct cross-sectional image is produced (Fig. 8-7D).

The LSFBP technique is further illustrated by the phantom study in Fig. 8-8. Even though some of the structure of the phantom is seen on the image without the filter, the defocused nature of the image limits the perception of the true structure as seen when the filter is added. The ACTA and Ohio-Nuclear scanners and later versions of the EMI scanner employ LSFBP or convolution reconstruction techniques to generate the reconstructed image.

The spatial resolution of a reconstructed LSFBP image depends on the range of frequencies in the filter function. The range is from zero to some upper limit or cutoff frequency, which establishes the highest frequency (e.g., highest spatial resolution) that will occur in the reconstructed image. The cutoff frequency is a critical parameter

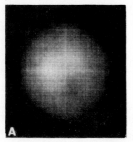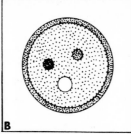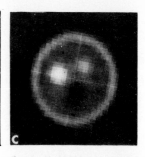

Fig. 8-8. Reconstructed images obtained from emission data (Chapter 7) using a Fourier-based algorithm with and without filter function. (A) Linear superposition of back projections, (B) cross section of actual object, and (C) linear superposition of filtered back projections.

and the value chosen will depend on detector resolution, linear and angular sampling resolution, and statistics. One would like to reconstruct with high spatial resolution, but as usual there are practical considerations, such as examination time, patient dose, and detector resolution and contrast, which pose certain limitations. If too high a cutoff frequency is used, the image will also contain oscillations and artifacts.

The level of statistical noise and artifacts can be significantly reduced by reducing the magnitude of the high-frequency components in the filter function. This in effect introduces spatial averaging or smoothing of the reconstructed image; thus, it also results in some loss of spatial resolution and contrast.

The LSFBP reconstruction technique exemplifies the general concepts of the Fourier-based algorithms. The various Fourier-based techniques may be operationally different but if done properly they all should yield the same reconstructed image. The relative merits of algebraic and Fourier-based reconstruction techniques are the subject of many discussions at this time and will not be dealt with here. However, a general conclusion is that Fourier-based techniques are faster in computation time and have lower computer memory (and/or magnetic disk and tape) requirements. Some comparisons of reconstructed images using algebraic and Fourier algorithms are presented by Shepp and Logan (*21*).

Sampling

Three important questions related to sampling are: (A) How many sampling points should be taken on the linear scan? (B) Over what total angle should data be taken? (C) How many discrete angles are necessary? These questions will be dealt with briefly.

The linear sampling requirements are derived from the sampling theorem (22). In general, the sampling theorem predicts that one must sample with a resolution at least twice as narrow as the object size to be recovered to obtain quantitative accuracy. In real (as opposed to ideal) circumstances, the linear sampling resolution should actually be three to four times narrower than the diameter of the smallest object to be recovered. For example, for a 6-mm-diam object, the sampling resolution should be less than about 2 mm. This does not mean that smaller objects will not be seen in the image, for indeed they will be if their contrast is high enough, but their values and shapes will be inaccurate (image contrast will be lower than object contrast).

To gather enough information to solve uniquely for the distribution of unknowns in the cross section, the angular scan should be performed over a full 180 deg. This is illustrated in Fig. 8-9 showing reconstructed images from scans taken over 90, 135, and 180 deg. On the scan performed over a 90-deg angle, the dark spots in the vertical direction run together and the horizontal ones have a depression between them. The situation is improved when the angle is increased 135 deg, but the true image is reconstructed only when the scan is carried out over a full 180 deg.

The number of discrete angles, m, at which linear scans should be performed is given by:

$$m \geq \pi\, D/2d \approx 1.5\, D/d \tag{8}$$

where D is the diameter of the cross section and d is the linear sampling resolution. Equation 8 was derived by Todd-Pokropek (23) from the projection theorem and indicates that angular sampling resolution should equal linear sampling resolution. Thus, if $\pi\, D/2$ is the length of the 180-deg arc of diam D (cross-sectional size), and if linear sampling is performed at intervals of d, then the number of angles is $\pi\, D/2$ divided by the interval length d. For example, if the linear sampling resolution d is 3 mm for a 200-mm-diam cross section, then:

$$m \geq \pi\, 200/(2 \times 3) = 105 \text{ angles.} \tag{9}$$

The first EMI scanner employed 3-mm linear sampling resolution with an 80×80 matrix. Thus the 180 angles taken at 1-deg steps satisfied Eq. 8 for a 200-mm-diam object. In the new version, which employs the 160×160 matrix, the 180 angular scans fall a little short of the value required by Eq. 8. If too few angles are taken, the full resolution and contrast are not recovered in the reconstructed image, and artifacts (star pattern) caused by gaps in the angular sampling may result. Spatial smoothing can be applied to remove these artifacts. However, this is done with the loss of some spatial resolution and contrast.

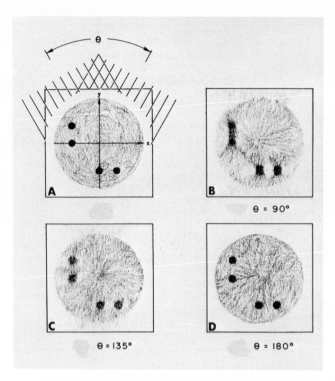

Fig. 8-9. Effect of angle through which data are taken on reconstructed image. (A) True object and scan angle, θ. (B) Scan through 90 deg. (C) Scan through 135 deg. (D) Scan through full 180 deg. Distortions are evident for scan angles less than 180 deg.

Physical Aspects

Certain physical aspects affect the quality of reconstructed CTT images. These include (A) the relatively small variations in the attenuation coefficients of different body fluids and tissues; (B) statistical quality of the image; (C) acceptance of scattered radiation; (D) the x-ray tube potential (kVp); (E) effect of the continuous energy distribution of the x-ray beam; and (F) the use of a water box surrounding the cross section examined.

Attenuation coefficients. Attenuation coefficients for 60-keV photons were measured for a number of fluids, soft tissues, and pathological samples (Table 8-1). It is clear that variations in either the transmitted intensity or the attenuation coefficients are extremely small, explaining why these structures are not normally seen on a plane film.

For the relatively high kVps (100–140) employed in CTT scanning, x-ray beam attenuation in soft tissue is mainly by Compton

TABLE 8-1. Attenuation of 60-keV Photons in Various Tissues and Fluids of the Brain

Tissue or fluids	Linear attenuation coefficient, μ (cm^{-1})	Percent transmitted photons through 1 cm relative to water
Fat*	0.1846	101.85
Water	0.2029	100.00
CSF	0.2063	99.67
Plasma	0.2072	99.58
Edematous tissue	0.2075	99.54
Necrotic tissue	0.2076	99.53
White matter	0.2088	99.48
Mixed brain tissue	0.2092	99.38
Grey matter	0.2106	99.24
Subdural hematoma	0.2112	99.18
Meningioma	0.2125	99.05
Whole blood†	0.2129	99.02
Clot	0.2209	98.23
RBC	0.2216	98.16
Metastasis, breast‡	0.2222	98.10

* Subcutaneous.
† Hematocrit of 40.
‡ Contained foci of calcium.

scattering, with a small but still significant contribution from photoelectric absorption. Attenuation by Compton scattering primarily reflects electron volume density (electrons/cm^3), which in turn depends on the physical density, ρ(gm/cm^3), and electron mass density (electrons/gm) of the attenuating material. Hydrogen content is a major factor affecting electron mass density because the electron mass density of hydrogen ($\sim 6 \times 10^{23}$ electrons/gm) is greater by about a factor of 2 than that of all other elements ($\sim 3 \times 10^{23}$ electrons/gm). Attenuation by photoelectric absorption depends strongly on effective atomic number (Z_{eff})^3 and small variations in Z_{eff} will produce significant changes in CTT-determined values of μ. This may be especially important if small amounts of high-Z elements such as calcium, phosphorus, or iron are present.

In CTT scanning of the brain, low values of μ (relative to white matter) probably reflect increased water content (low electron density), or lipid content (low electron density and low Z), while high values probably reflect increased cellular density, blood content, or high-Z elements (Table 8-1). Edematous brain tissue, for example, has a higher water content than normal brain and its relatively low value of μ may reflect the low electron density of water compared to normal brain tissue. Also, the low atomic number and electron density of adipose tissue may explain why its attenuation coefficient is lower than that of water by about 10% (Table 8-1). This figure is consistent with EMI values of -30 ($\mu \sim 6\%$ lower than water) that we have observed for retro-orbital fat. The value of μ for chronic subdural hematoma shown in Table 8-1 is close to that of grey matter. This may explain reported instances in which this lesion was not detected by CTT scanning (24, 25). We have found that at a later stage chronic subdural hematomas show values even lower than normal brain tissue, approximating those of cerebrospinal fluid. Chronic subdural hematomas are known to undergo a progressive decrease of their content of iron (high Z) pigment. On the other hand, a fresh blood clot has a high content of iron pigment and a high density, which probably produce the high value of μ (Table 8-1). There are obviously many other factors that can produce the variations of μ in soft tissues, and much more information is needed in this area.

Statistics. The small differences in μ and the small sizes of the different structures in the brain produce correspondingly small variations in transmitted beam intensity and require that sufficient photons be collected to obtain statistical precision to a fraction of a percent. The total number of photons recorded for an EMI image is about 2×10^9. This has been shown (21, 26) to yield a statistical precision of better than 0.5% (1 s.d.) for the 3-mm resolution in the 80×80 reconstruction array of the first EMI scanners. However, in the newer version with the 160×160 array, statistical mottle is more apparent in the image. Statistical variations can be reduced by image smoothing, but this results in loss of resolution.

Improvements in spatial resolution in CTT scanning require drastic increases in radiation dose to the patient and in examination times. It has been shown (27) that in reconstruction tomography the total number of photons, N, required to obtain an image with a given level of statistical noise per resolution element is inversely related to the third power of resolution, Δx, in the cross-sectional plane, $N \propto 1/\Delta x^3$. This is in contrast to the situation in conventional two-dimensional imaging, e.g., radionuclide scanning, for which $N \propto 1/\Delta x^2$. Furthermore, in transmission scanning, the width of the exposed detector area, and thus detector sensitivity, are inversely related to Δx. Therefore, for a given photon flux or source strength, the total examination time, T, is inversely related to the fourth power of resolution, $T \propto 1/\Delta x^4$. Thus in reconstruction tomography, if resolution in the cross-sectional plane is to be increased by a factor of 2 for the same source strength and statistical noise per resolution element, the number of photons recorded for the image must be increased by a factor of 8 and the examination time by a factor of 16. For example, these required increases could be achieved as follows: (A) twice as many linear scans (at half the angular separations); (B) twice as many readings per linear scan; and (C) four times the measuring time per measurement. Because of the reduced detector sensitivity, the last factor will result in only twice as many photons per measurement. Note that the radiation dose, D, to the examined cross section increases only by a factor of 8, i.e., $D \propto 1/\Delta x^3$. This is because while twice as many measurements are recorded per scan, each element of tissue is still measured (irradiated) only once per linear scan.

These conclusions apply to resolution, Δx, in the cross-sectional plane, but the same reasoning can be applied to the resolution in thickness, Δy, of the cross-sectional plane. For radiation dose, one obtains $D \propto 1/\Delta x^3 \, \Delta y$, and for examination time, $T \propto 1/\Delta x^4 \, \Delta y^2$. Therefore, if both the thickness and cross-sectional resolution are to be improved by a factor of 2 for the same source strength and statistical noise per resolution element, the radiation dose to the examined tissue must be increased by a factor of 16, and examination time by a factor of 64. This assumes that twice as many sections would be scanned so that one still obtains a complete examination of the organ.

These considerations indicate that there are certain limitations on the resolution obtainable in practical CTT scanning systems. One could alleviate the examination time requirements somewhat by using a multiple detector system or by increasing the photon flux (higher tube current or multiple tubes). However, neither of these approaches would have any effect on patient dose.

Scattered radiation. Two of the more important aspects of CTT scanning are the reduced amounts of scatter obtained with a narrow-beam scanning technique and replacement of x-ray film by a quantitative radiation detector. It has been shown (28) that, in a conventional full-field radiographic examination of a 25-cm-thick water phantom using 100 kVp without a grid, the scatter to primary ratio is approximately 2:1 for a 10 × 10-cm field, while for a 30 × 30-cm field the ratio is 7:1. If a 100 line/in. grid (grid ratio, 8) is employed, these ratios are reduced to 1:1 and 3:1. This indicates that in conventional full-field radiography the amount of scattered radiation may be substantially greater than the amount of primary radiation. This is probably one of the largest single factors limiting the contrast obtainable by conventional radiography.

The narrow-beam scanning technique and the full-field examination were compared by taking a radiograph of a plastic step wedge on a water box and then scanning the same water box and step wedge with a 3 × 3-mm beam of x-rays and a collimated NaI(Tl) detector. The wedge steps reduced the transmitted primary beam intensity by 16%, 9%, 4%, 2%, 1%, and 0.5% relative to water. On the radiograph, only the 16%, 9%, 4%, and, with some imagination, the 2% step could be seen whereas with the narrow-beam scanning technique all the steps were detected (Fig. 8-10). Thus the narrow-beam scanning technique exhibits high inherent contrast and also validates one of the

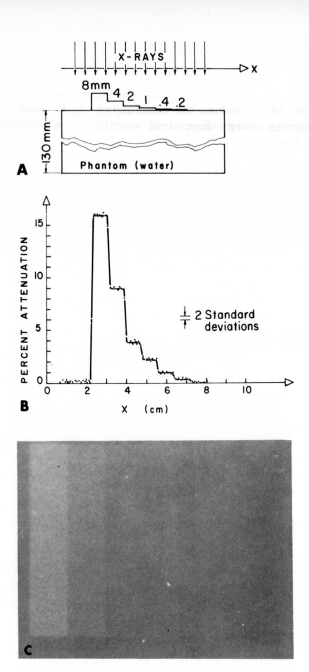

Fig. 8-10. Comparison of contrast of plastic step wedge obtained by radiographic and narrow-beam scanning techniques with 80-kVp x-ray beam. (A) Plastic step wedge was positioned on top of 13-cm-thick water phantom. Steps were designed to reduce beam intensity by 16%, 9%, 4%, 2%, 1%, and 0.5%. (B) Narrow-beam scanning profile obtained with 3 × 3-mm x-ray beam and NaI(Tl) detector. All steps are detected. (C) Radiograph obtained with 100 line/in. grid (grid ratio, 8). Only 16%, 9%, and 4% steps are seen.

assumptions of the algorithm, namely that very little scattered radiation reaches the detector.

High kVp in CTT. A high kVp technique is used in CTT scanning for three reasons: (A) to produce a high transmitted beam flux at the detector; (B) to reduce the contrast of skull relative to brain; and (C) to minimize energy-dependent variations in attenuation coefficients.

A high transmitted beam flux is necessary because of the low geometric efficiency of the detector system with a narrow-beam technique, coupled with the requirements for a high level of statistical precision needed to detect small variations in soft-tissue attenuation. The use of relatively high kVp provides a high transmission flux, first, because the x-ray tube output intensity increases as $(kVp)^{3*}$ and, second, because overall beam attenuation is less for higher energy photons.

It is desirable to reduce the contrast differential between skull and soft tissues for two reasons. First, small variations of skull thickness could mask small variations in soft-tissue attenuation and, second, any large abrupt change in attenuation tends to produce artifacts in regions of the reconstructed CTT image near the abrupt change (21). This could reduce the sensitivity of the technique for regions near bone.

Problems arising from the energy-dependent nature of attenuation coefficients are discussed in the next section. It suffices to say at this time that variations of attenuation coefficients with energy become smaller as the beam energy is increased.

A negative aspect of using a high kVp is that differences in soft-tissue attenuation coefficients also decrease with increasing x-ray energy. This factor must be balanced against the above factors to produce the optimum image.

Polychromatic x-ray beam and the water box. One of the tacit assumptions of CTT scanning is that the x-ray beam is monochromatic. Specifically, one assumes that the attenuation coefficient of a cell within the cross section is the same when measured from all possible angles through the head. With the polychromatic beam from an x-ray tube, however, the transmitted energy spectrum (or average beam energy) and, therefore, the measured attenuation coefficients may change with viewing angle, depending on the total thickness of tissue traversed, the thickness of bone in the beam, etc. This effect is known as "beam hardening" and is characteristic of polychromatic beams. As pointed out by McCullough, et al (30) in CTT scanning one

---

* Some texts have indicated that x-ray output intensity increases as $(kVp)^2$. However, this refers to the intensity of the beam leaving the target. For a heavily filtered beam outside the tube, intensity is proportional to $(kVp)^3$ (29). The dc detection mode of CTT scanning measures intensity (number of photons times energy) so $(kVp)^3$ is applicable.

might expect to find possible variations in the calculated attenuation coefficient for a cell containing a particular substance, depending on exactly where the cell was located in the cross section, and on the location of other structures such as bones and air spaces. Therefore, the problem deserves careful evaluation.

It has been suggested by some authors that problems related to the polychromatic nature of the x-ray beam could be eliminated by using radionuclide sources. However, it should be noted that the photon flux from an x-ray tube operating at 120 kVp, 30 mA is equivalent to about 15,000 Ci of a radionuclide source. Furthermore, for high spatial resolution this must be concentrated into an area of a few square millimeters, which is not possible with radionuclides of reasonable half-life. Therefore, x-ray tubes will probably continue to be used for CTT scanning.

We investigated the transmission of 120-kVp x-ray beams through various thicknesses of plastic and bone. On a semi-log graph (Fig. 8-11) the curve for plastic was a straight line over most of the 0–25-cm thickness range. The small deviation in the initial part of the curve was removed when an additional 4-mm aluminum filtration was added. This produced a straight line which fit a monoexponential curve from 0 to 25 cm with a correlation coefficient, r = 0.999. The same measurements for 0–5 cm of bone did not produce a straight line (Fig. 8-11) even with the added 4-mm aluminum filtration, indicating significant beam hardening is possible in bone.

One purpose of the water box and constant path length used in some CTT scanners, e.g., the EMI scanner, is to minimize variations in the energy spectrum of the transmitted beam (and therefore in attenuation coefficients) that might result from passing the beam through different thicknesses of tissue. Removal of the water box and the possible effects on accuracy have therefore become points of controversy. Mathematically, the problem may be evaluated as follows.* Consider a thickness, x, of water containing a thickness, Δx, of some other material. For an x-ray beam with a continuous energy distribution, the total transmitted beam intensity, I_n, is given by:

$$I_n = \int_0^{E_{max}} I_0(E)e^{-\mu_w(E)x}\, e^{-(\mu_i(E)-\mu_w(E))\Delta x}\, dE \qquad (10)$$

where $I_0(E)$ describes the incident intensity spectrum and $\mu_w(E)$ and $\mu_i(E)$ are the attenuation coefficients for water and the added material, respectively. The intensity spectrum of the reference beam may be written as:

$$I_R(E) = I_0(E)e^{-\mu_R(E)R} \qquad (11)$$

where $I_0(E)$ is the intensity spectrum from the tube, R is the thickness

---

* A similar derivation was presented by McCullough, et al (30).

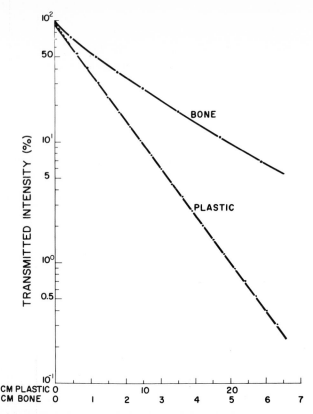

Fig. 8-11. Transmitted x-ray intensity vs. thickness of plastic or bone. A 4 × 4-mm beam and a 130-kVp technique with 2 mm or 6 mm of added Al filtration were employed (see text). Solid line represents monoexponential curve. Dashed line represents deviation from monoexponential from 0–3 cm for plastic.

of the reference beam absorber, and $\mu_R(E)$ is the attenuation coefficient of the reference beam material. Thus, Eq. 10 can be written:

$$I_n = \int_0^{E_{max}} I_R(E)e^{-(\mu_w(E)x-\mu_R(E)R)}\,e^{-(\mu_i(E)-\mu_w(E))\Delta x}dE. \qquad (12)$$

Although $\mu_i(E)$ and $\mu_w(E)$ may show an appreciable energy dependence, the difference term is in most cases more slowly varying over the range of energies in the beam (primarily 40–120 keV). In fact, for soft tissues, the assumption that $\mu_i(E) - \mu_w(E)$ is constant is reasonable because most of the interactions are by Compton scattering. Therefore, $\mu_i(E) - \mu_w(E)$ reflects a difference in electron densities of tissue and water and is independent of photon energy. This assumption becomes less valid as the fraction of interactions occurring by photoelectric absorption increases. For materials containing heavy elements such as bone the assumption might not be valid because of the strong energy dependence of photoelectric absorption and the predominance of photoelectric absorption in high-Z elements.

If it is assumed that the difference is constant, we may write:

$$I_n = e^{-(\mu_i - \mu_w)\Delta x} \int_0^{E_{max}} I_R(E) e^{-(\mu_w(E)x - \mu_R(E)R)} dE. \qquad (13)$$

One would like to write the integral in this equation as I_R, the total intensity of the reference beam, times perhaps some constant factor for all of the measurements in a CTT scan. For scans made with a water box this can in fact be done, because $\mu_w(E)x - \mu_R(E)R$ is constant for all scans, and furthermore it is a small term since the reference beam attenuator thickness is chosen to give the same total attenuation as a water box of thickness x. Thus, Eq. 12 reduces to:

$$I_n = I_R e^{-(\mu_i - \mu_w)\Delta x} \qquad (14)$$

and one may then proceed to solve the problem as if the beam were monochromatic, as represented by Eq. 5.

For scans made without the water box this is no longer the case because the thickness, x, is not constant for all measurements and therefore the integral in Eq. 13 is not related by a constant factor to I_R, the reference beam intensity. Corrective techniques could be incorporated into the reconstruction algorithm to compensate for this effect. Unfortunately, not enough is known at the present time about the performance characteristics of scanners not employing the water box to state whether or not this represents a real problem. However, the ACTA-scan example shown in Fig. 11-3 is suggestive of possible difficulties.

The water box serves a number of other purposes. One requirement of a CTT system is that it must take tens of thousands of transmission readings accurately without any variations in detection efficiency. This is facilitated by the water box, which limits the dynamic range over which the detector must operate and therefore reduces nonlinearity and instability problems. For example, x-ray transmission intensity varies by factors of 7 and 70, respectively, in a scan of the head with and without the water box. Values of μ vary between those of air and bone without the water box, as compared to water and bone with the water box.

Large changes in the attenuation coefficients such as at the boundary between air, skull, and soft tissue produce artifacts (oscillations in the image).* The artifacts are greatest near the boundary.

---

* These oscillations produced a decrease in values near the interior of the skull in the first version of the EMI scanner and were thought to preclude the detection of subdural hematomas. They also caused the distortion of the image in patients with clips. These problems have been reduced to some degree in the new EMI scanners by the use of a convolution algorithm instead of the algebraic technique. The ACTA and Ohio-Nuclear scanners also use a convolution reconstruction technique.

Their magnitude depends on the size of the change at the boundary and on the algorithm. In general, the larger the change at a boundary the larger is the artifact produced. This suggests that the level of artifacts should be less with the water box than without it. Various correction schemes could be applied to reduce these artifacts. However, it is difficult to further evaluate problems associated with the removal of the water box in the commercial systems at the present time because of the limited information available on their CTT systems.

Performance Characteristics

Some performance characteristics of CTT scanning were evaluated on an EMI scanner using a Fourier-based algorithm and a 160×160 display matrix. Both 80×80 and 160×160 numerical printouts were used to evaluate quantitative accuracy. Phantom studies were carried out to assess accuracy, spatial variations of μ, effect of varying the object size and contrast, orientation of object in the examined cross section, and artifacts caused by the skull and by motion.

The phantom used in this work was a water-filled plastic cylinder about the size of a human head. Inside the cylinder were partitions onto which could be mounted up to nine plastic rods of different sizes and compositions. The phantom was scanned with the cylinders perpendicular to the cross-sectional slice. Most of the EMI scan images to be presented show that some air bubbles were trapped in the phantom. These were not removed because air is also present in scans on patients, trapped in the hair. In any case none of our measurements indicated a significant ($>0.5\%$) difference in results for relatively small (1–2 cc) amounts of trapped air.

Accuracy. The accuracy of the system was assessed by placing different types of 18-mm-diam plastic rods in the phantom. The types of plastic, physical density, electron density, effective atomic number, and the measured EMI number are listed in Table 8-2. The EMI number was determined by calculating the mean value of an area corresponding to an interior 12-mm-diam section of the rod from the numerical printout in the 80×80 array. Data for water are also given in Table 8-2. The EMI number for water was calculated from a 3×3-cm section of the image representing water in the phantom. The value for water on the EMI scale is approximately zero. Positive and negative numbers represent attenuation coefficients greater and less than water, respectively. An EMI number of 5 units corresponds to a 1% change in the attenuation coefficient relative to water (~ 0.002 cm^{-1}). These results are in good agreement with some results reported earlier by McCullough, et al (*30*).

TABLE 8-2   EMI Scanner Values for Different Types of Plastics*

Material	EMI number† (mean ± σ)			Density (gm/cc)	Electron density (electrons/cc) × 10²³	Effective atomic number, Z_{eff}‡
Teflon	441.0	± 15.1	(27.6)	2.16	6.30	8.43
Delrin	183.9	± 2.2	(2.9)	1.42	4.55	6.95
Nylon	44.7	± 1.9	(2.7)	1.14	3.77	6.12
Water	−0.2	± 0.2	(1.5)	1.00	3.34	7.42
Polystyrene	−14.1	± 0.8	(2.2)	1.06	3.43	5.69
Polyethylene (high density)	−38.6	± 1.6	(2.5)	0.96	3.29	5.44
Polyethylene (low density)	−51.8	± 2.1	(2.9)	0.92	3.17	5.44

* Taken from the numerical printout for an 80 × 80 array.
† Mean and standard deviation for multiple measurements. Numbers in parentheses are standard deviations of individual grid element values in a single measurement.
‡ Effective atomic number was calculated in accordance with Mayneord (31).

Means and standard deviations for single and multiple measurements are also given in Table 8-2. A large part of the error for Teflon resulted from artifacts caused by its large discontinuity with the surrounding water, which produces oscillations and an apparent depression in attenuation at the center of the rod.

It is interesting to note that, while polystyrene has both an electron density and physical density greater than water, its EMI number is negative relative to water. If all the x-ray interactions were by Compton scattering, it should have an attenuation coefficient greater than water, because the Compton interactions are dependent on electron density. We attribute this result to the lower probability for photoelectric interactions in polystyrene resulting from its lower effective atomic number. Because of the Z^3 dependence of photoelectric interactions, it only requires that about 3% of the photons interact through the photoelectric process to compensate for the differences in electron and physical densities and yield the measured value of −14.1 for polystyrene relative to water. This indicates that the attenuation coefficients of materials in the body as presently measured by CTT scanning depend on both electron density and effective atomic number.

The mean value for water was measured to be −0.2 with a standard deviation of ±1.5 EMI units for a single grid element in the 80 × 80 array. This represents a system noise level of ± 0.3% ($\Delta\mu \approx 0.0006$ cm⁻¹), which is a little better than the value quoted by EMI of ± 0.5% (3).

The standard deviation per grid element as measured with a water phantom increased in going from the 80 × 80 array to the

160 × 160 array (Table 8-3). Transmitted intensity was also varied by a factor of 3.2 by adjusting the collimator size and the scan time. As seen in Table 8-3, the decrease in noise level followed the pattern predicted from the increasing number of transmitted photons (square root of the number of transmitted photons). This indicates that the major contribution to noise is from photon statistics and not from the algorithm or the radiation detector and associate electronics. Thus the information obtainable from the EMI scanner appears to be photon limited.

These factors are also illustrated in Fig. 8-12 showing EMI scan images of a water phantom for different total numbers of photons recorded in the image. The left-hand image is comparable to what is obtained in many clinical situations, representing a 13-mm slice thickness at 120 kVp and 33 mA.

When the phantom was surrounded with a 6-mm-thick sheet of Teflon to simulate the skull, somewhat larger standard deviations were obtained, probably the result of a 30% decrease in the photon flux.

Spatial variations in μ. When 18-mm-diam polystyrene rods were placed at the 12, 9, 6, and 3 o'clock and the center positions in the examined cross section, variations of less than 2.6 EMI units (0.5% in μ of water) were observed in the measured attenuation. This indicates that the system yields values of μ for cerebral tissues that do not depend on position, which is in agreement with the data reported by McCullough, et al (30).

Effect of object size on contrast. Polystyrene rods of 18-, 10-, 6-, 3-, and 1-mm diam were placed in the water phantom and scanned (Fig. 8-13). All the rods were seen in the reconstructed image with the exception of the 1-mm-diam rod. The EMI number for the 18-mm-diam rod was -13.9 ($\mu \sim 2.8\%$ less than water). The average values for the 10-, 6-, and 3-mm-diam rods were -13.3, -11.2, and -8, respectively, corresponding to 96%, 81%, and 58% relative to the value for the 18-mm-diam rod. This indicates a decrease in quantitative accuracy and image contrast as object size is decreased for a fixed object contrast of 3% less than water.

Figure 8-14 shows the EMI image of the phantom with Nylon ($\mu \sim 9\%$ greater than water) rods of 10-, 6-, and 3-mm diam; polystyrene ($\mu \sim 3\%$ less than water) rods of 10-, 6-, and 3-mm diam; Teflon ($\mu \sim 90\%$ greater than water) rods of 3- and 1-mm diam; and a Delrin ($\mu \sim 37\%$ greater than water) rod of 1-mm diam. All of the rods are seen in the image. The high contrast of Delrin and Teflon (Teflon is about the same as bone) allows observation of a 1-mm-diam object, although it appeared in the image to have a size of about 3 mm. Image contrasts for the 1-mm-diam Teflon and Delrin rods were only about 5% of the true values.

TABLE 8-3. Standard Deviation of EMI Values for Water as a Function of Array Size and Number of Transmitted Photons Recorded

Collimator size × scan time (mm × min)	Relative number of transmitted photons	Standard deviation for water (EMI units)				
		Experimental		Predicted*		
		80 × 80	160 × 160	80 × 80	160 × 160	
8 × 4.5†	1.0	± 1.64	± 2.56	± 1.54	± 2.32	
13 × 4.5	1.6	± 1.25	± 1.86	± 1.21	± 1.83	
13 × 9	3.2	± 0.86	± 1.30	± 0.86	± 1.30	

* From relative number of transmitted photons.
† Since the phantom did not contain a skull, the 4.5-min scan time and 8-mm slice thickness give results comparable to a 4.5-min scan time with a 13-mm slice thickness for an average head.

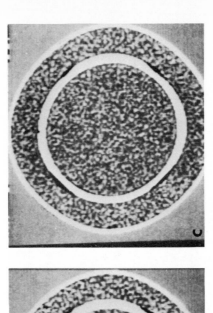

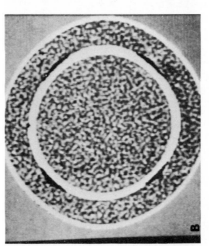

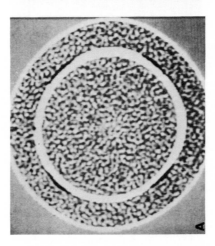

Fig. 8-12. EMI image of water-filled plastic phantom illustrating variations in noise level with total number of detected photons. (A) Relative number of photons = 1. (B) Relative number of photons = 1.6. (C) Relative number of photons = 3.2. A is comparable to clinical situation for 13-mm slice thickness at 120 kVp, 33 mA.

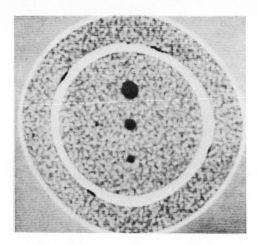

Fig. 8-13. EMI image of polystyrene rods of 1–18-mm diam in water phantom. The rods in center column, from top to bottom, were 18-, 10-, and 6-mm diam. The 3-mm rod was at left and 1-mm rod (not seen in image) was at right. Two large white rings are plastic phantom and plastic retaining cone of EMI scanner. Window level was from −25 to +15 EMI units.

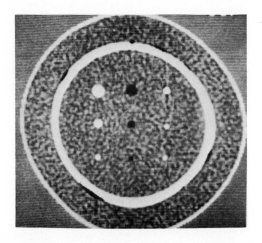

Fig. 8-14. EMI image of plastic rods of different compositions and sizes. Left: Nylon (μ 9% greater than H_2O) rods (top to bottom) 10-, 6-, and 3-mm diam. Center: polystyrene (μ 3% less than H_2O) rods of 10-, 6-, and 3-mm diam. Right: Teflon (μ 90% greater than H_2O) rods 3- and 1-mm diam and Delrin (μ 37% greater than H_2O) rod 1-mm diam. Window level was from −30 to +20 EMI units.

Orientation of the object in the examined cross section. For all of the scans described above, the objects had lengths greater than the 13-mm slice thickness and were placed perpendicular to the cross section. For Fig. 8-15, short pieces of 10-, 6-, and 3-mm-diam poly-

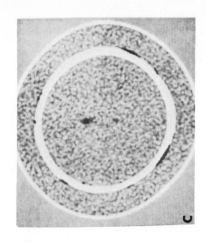

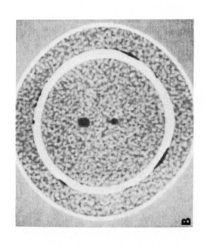

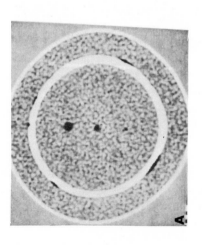

Fig. 8-15. EMI images of polystyrene rods perpendicular and tilted by 40 deg to scanning plane. (A) Images of 10-, 6-, and 3-mm-diam rods perpendicular to scanning plane. (B) Images of tilted 10- and 6-mm-diam rods. (C) Images of tilted 6- and 3-mm-diam rods. Window level was from −25 to +15 EMI units.

styrene rods were positioned in the phantom and tilted 40 deg so that only a portion of the thickness of the slice contained the rods. The 10- and 6-mm-diam rods in the tilted position were seen with about a 10–20% decrease in image contrast, which is consistent with the 10–20% decrease in occupancy of the tilted rods in the thickness of the slice. The 3-mm-diam rod which had an average EMI value of −8 in the perpendicular position was barely discernible from noise. This illustrates the loss of contrast for small objects in the relatively thick (13 and 8 mm) slice employed in the EMI scanner and the importance of including thickness of the slice as a part of the system resolution. Reduction of slice thickness may improve resolution, but it also reduces the transmitted x-ray intensity, thereby increasing statistical noise in the image; it also increases the number of slices required for a total examination. These factors must be carefully weighed against the improvement in overall spatial resolution.

Effects of skull and patient motion. Large discontinuities in attenuation coefficients such as between the skull and soft tissue produce artifacts in the reconstructed image near the discontinuity. This artifact is usually seen as a negative undershoot near the skull. As discussed by Shepp and Logan (*21*), Fourier reconstruction techniques reduce this artifact as compared to algebraic techniques. Figure 8-16 is a reconstructed image of a skull in a water phantom obtained with the EMI scanner using a Fourier-based algorithm. Undershoot, which would have appeared as a dark shadow at the skull-water interface, is not seen in the image. It should be pointed out that for metal clips the discontinuity is so large that artifacts are produced throughout the image even with the Fourier-based algorithm presently employed by EMI. One method for reducing the artifacts from large discontinuities is to employ spatial smoothing in the reconstruction algorithm, but this is done with some loss of spatial resolution and contrast.

The importance of immobilizing the patient during a CTT examination is demonstrated in Fig. 8-17, showing EMI images of a patient with and without motion. At the Mallinckrodt Institute approximately 2% of the patient images are discarded and another 15% contain significant artifacts because of excessive patient motion.

Future Developments in CTT Scanning

Reconstruction algorithms employed in CTT scanning have been described to illustrate the basic principles of the different techniques. While we have made no effort to compare directly algebraic and Fourier reconstruction algorithms, it is fair to say that if done properly they should produce images of comparable quality. A distinct advantage of the Fourier-based techniques is their shorter computa-

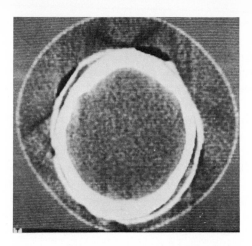

Fig. 8-16. EMI image of human skull in water phantom. Two outer rings are plastic phantom holding skull and plastic retaining cone in the EMI water box. Dark spots around plastic phantom are from air trapped between rubber cap and phantom. Window level was from −37.5 to +37.5 EMI units.

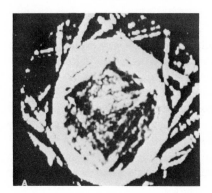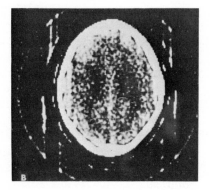

Fig. 8-17. EMI images of patient with (A) and without (B) patient motion. Window level was from −5 to +25 EMI units.

tion time, one of the primary reasons that newer CTT scanners all employ this technique. As scan times decrease with newer devices, this factor will become even more important, and computations will probably be performed in hard-wired circuits rather than with the standard programmed computer to allow reconstructed images to be generated in a matter of seconds for array sizes of about 160 × 160.

Major changes in CTT scanners that are likely to occur in the future will result from changes in the detector systems (new detector systems such as gas ionization or proportional counters), use of large multiple detector arrays, and changes in the type of scanning motion employed. These changes will shorten the examination time and improve spatial resolution. Examination times can be decreased by increasing the number of detectors and the size of the beam up to the point at which the entire cross-sectional plane is examined at one time. A possible problem with this technique is that scattered radiation will also increase as the size and number of collimated x-ray beams are increased, possibly degrading image contrast. However, longer detector collimators could be employed to minimize the acceptance of scattered radiation without a large decrease in primary beam intensity.

Improving spatial resolution will be a difficult task because of its strong relationship to the number of photons recorded, patient dose, and examination time (increasing the number of detectors and x-ray beam size shortens examination time, but does not affect dose). For example, if the x-ray beam dimensions were reduced from 3×13 mm to 0.5×0.5 mm, and data were reconstructed in a 320×320 array to give a resolution in all three dimensions of about 0.5 mm, the total dose would be increased by a factor of approximately 5,600, and examination time by a factor of approximately 875,000 (for the same number of detectors) over present levels. These factors place certain limitations on the possibilities for improving the resolution of CTT techniques.

Variations in attenuation coefficients (μ) of soft tissue and fluids with the present CTT scanners result from differences in both electron density (Compton interactions) and atomic number (photoelectric interactions). Much more information is needed on the correlation between physiological and pathological factors that produce changes in attenuation to evaluate the potential for differential diagnosis by CTT scanning.

The technique of transaxial transmission reconstruction tomography is without doubt one of the most significant advances for noninvasive examination of the brain in the past 50 years. However, the technique itself is as important as its specific application to studies of the brain or other parts of the body. Reconstruction techniques have previously been successfully applied to the field of radionuclide imaging (Chapters 4, 5, and 7) and will find other applications in medicine in the future.

Acknowledgments

We thank H. Huang, J. R. Cox, and D. Snyder for many helpful discussions. This work was partially supported by NIH Grants 5 PO1 HL13851 and 1 RO1 HL15423, and by NIH Fellowship 1 FO3 GM55196-01.

References

1. HODES PH, DeMOOR J, ERNST R: Body section radiography: Fundamentals. *Radiol Clin North Am* 1: 229–244, 1963

2. LITTLETON JT, RUMBAUGH CL, WINTER FS: Polydirectional body section roentgenography. A new diagnostic method. *Am J Roentgenol Radium Ther Nucl Med* 89: 1179–1193, 1963

3. LITTLETON JT: A phantom method to evaluate the clinical effectiveness of a tomographic device. *Am J Roentgenol Radium Ther Nucl Med* 108: 847–856, 1970

4. ANGER H: Multiplane tomographic scanner. In *Tomographic Imaging in Nuclear Medicine,* Freedman GS, ed, New York, Society of Nuclear Medicine, 1973, pp 2–15

5. HOUNSFIELD GN: Computerized transverse axial scanning (tomography): Part 1. Description of system. *Br J Radiol* 46: 1016–1022, 1973

6. HOUNSFIELD GN: A method of and apparatus for examination of a body by radiation such as x or gamma radiation. London, The Patent Office, Patent specification 1283915, 1972

7. LEDLEY RS, DICHIRO G, LUESSENHOP AJ, et al: Computerized transaxial x-ray tomography of the human body. *Science* 186: 207–212, 1974

8. GORDON R, HERMAN GT: Three dimensional reconstruction from projections: a review of algorithms. *Int Rev Cytol* 38: 111–151, 1974

9. KUHL DE, EDWARDS RQ: Image separation radioisotope scanning. *Radiology* 80: 653–662, 1963

10. KUHL, DE, EDWARDS RQ, RICCI AR, et al: Quantitative section scanning using orthogonal tangent correction. *J Nucl Med* 14: 196–200, 1973

11. GORDON R, BENDER R, HERMAN GT: Algebraic reconstruction technique. *J Theor Biol* 29: 471–481, 1970

12. GILBERT P: Iterative methods for the reconstruction of three-dimensional objects from projections. *J Theor Biol* 36: 105–117, 1972

13. MEYERS M: Tomography. Symposium of the British Nuclear Medicine Society, London, April, 1973

14. BRACEWELL R, RIDDLE A: Inversion of fan-beam scans in radio astronomy. *Astrophys J* 150: 427–434, 1967

15. TRETIAK OJ, EDEN M, SIMON W: Internal structures from x-ray images. In *Proceedings of 8th International Conference in Medical and Biological Engineering,* Chicago, Session 12-1, 1969

16. CORMACK AM: Representation of a function by its line integrals, with some radiological applications. *J Appl Phys* 34: 2722–2727, 1963

17. CORMACK AM: Reconstruction densities from their projections, with applications in radiological physics. *Phys Med Biol* 18: 195–207, 1973

18. CHESLER DA: Three-dimensional activity distributions from multiple positron scintigraphs. *J Nucl Med* 12: 347–348, 1971

19. TODD-POKROPEK AE: The formation and display of section scans. In *Proceedings of Symposium of American Congress of Radiology,* 1971, Amsterdam, Excerpta Medica, 1972, p 542

20. CHO AH, AHN A, TSAI C: Computer algorithms and detector electronics for the transmission x-ray tomography. *IEEE Trans Nucl Sci* NS-21, 1, 218–227, 1974

21. SHEPP LA, LOGAN BF: Some insights into the Fourier reconstruction of a head section, *IEEE Trans Nucl Sci* NS-21, 21–43, 1974

22. HANCOCK JC: *An Introduction to the Principles of Communication Theory.* New York, McGraw-Hill, 1951, p 18

23. TODD-POKROPEK AE: Tomography and the reconstruction of images from their projections. In *Proceedings of the Third International Conference on Data Handling and Image Processing Scintigraphy,* Metz C, ed, Boston, 1973: to be published

24. PAXTON CR, AMBROSE J: The EMI scanner. A brief review of the first 650 patients. *Br J Radiol* 47: 530–565, 1974

25. DAVIS DO, PRESSMAN BD: Computerized tomography of the brain. *Radiol Clin North Am* 12: 297–313, 1974

26. HUANG S, SNYDER D, COX J: Personal communication, 1974

27. CHESLER DA, ARONOW S, CORRELLE JE, et al: Statistical properties and simulation studies of transverse section algorithms. In *Workshop on Reconstruction Tomography in Diagnostic Radiology and Nuclear Medicine,* April, 1975, San Juan, Puerto Rico, Baltimore, University Park Press: to be published

28. TER-POGOSSIAN MM, PHELPS ME, HOFFMAN EJ, et al: The extraction of the yet unused wealth of information in diagnostic radiology. *Radiology* 113: 515–520, 1974

29. HOFFMAN EJ, PHELPS ME: Production of monoenergetic x-rays from 8 to 87 keV. *Phys Med Biol* 19: 19–35, 1974

30. McCULLOUGH EC, BAKER JL, HOUSER OW, et al: An evaluation of the quantitative and radiation features of a scanning x-ray transverse axial tomograph: the EMI scanner. *Radiology* 111: 709–715, 1974

31. MAYNEORD WV: The significance of the roentgen. *Acta Int Union Cancer* 2: 271, 1937

Chapter 9

Clinical Comparison of Radionuclide Brain Imaging and Computerized Transmission Tomography, I

Mokhtar Gado, R. Edward Coleman, and Philip O. Alderson

Several reports have predicted that computerized transaxial tomography (CTT scanning) would have a significant impact on the utilization of other neuroradiological techniques including radionuclide brain imaging (1-3). Although some reports have concluded that CTT scanning is more sensitive for detecting brain lesions than radionuclide imaging (1-4), they have not been based on a paired comparison of the two techniques. The purpose of this study is to compare the results and accuracy of both techniques in different pathological conditions.

Clinical Material

Our study population was drawn from 714 patients evaluated both by radionuclide imaging with an Anger camera (pertechnetate brain scanning or cisternography) and by CTT scanning with an EMI scanner during the period February to November, 1974. Approximately one-half of the EMI studies were performed with an 80 × 80 matrix and the other half with a 160 × 160 matrix. Among these patients, 362 had both normal radionuclide studies and normal CTT scans and were not included in the study. We also excluded 203 patients who showed evidence of cerebral atrophy or hydrocephalus on the CTT scan but who were not evaluated by cisternography. Our study group thus included 149 patients. These were divided into three categories based on the final diagnosis as follows: (A) intracranial masses, cysts, and vascular malformations (76 patients); (B) cerebrovascular disease (29 patients); and (C) cerebral atrophy or communicating hydrocephalus (44 patients). The results in each of these categories will be presented and analyzed separately.

Intracranial Masses, Cysts, and Vascular Malformations

Methods. In patients with suspected subdural hematomas, arteriovenous malformations, hydrocephalus, or cystic hemispheric lesions, a rapid sequence study was performed using a bolus injection of 15–20 mCi of ^{99m}Tc-pertechnetate. Each patient received $KClO_4$ prior to the study. Anterior or posterior projections were chosen on the basis of pertinent neurological signs and symptoms. The study was considered normal if there was symmetrical carotid activity, symmetrical arterial flow to the hemispheres, and no area of increased or decreased vascularity.

Immediately following the rapid sequence study, a 400,000-count image was obtained with the patient in the same position. This image aided in assessing the vascularity of lesions and in determining head shape in the projection used for the rapid sequence study. It was particularly helpful for evaluating those cases in which asymmetrical flow seen on the rapid sequence study led to consideration of a possible subdural hematoma.

Static brain images were obtained approximately 30 min after injection using a scintillation camera with a high resolution parallel-hole collimator. They included anterior, posterior, and both lateral views. Delayed images (2–4 hr) were obtained if the initial views were nondiagnostic or if indicated by clinical history (e.g., possible subdural hematoma). Occasionally, additional projections such as a vertex view and converging or pinhole collimator view of the posterior fossa were obtained.

When an abnormality was detected by radionuclide brain imaging, the morphology and site of the lesion were recorded. The size of the lesion was graded subjectively. If it involved less than 10% of the hemisphere it was considered small. If it involved 10–25% of the hemisphere it was considered moderate in size. If it involved greater than 25% of the hemisphere it was termed a large lesion. Lesion intensity was graded on a scale of 1–4 by comparing the lesion activity with that of the sagittal sinus. A grade 1 lesion was barely visible, a grade 2 lesion was easily seen but less intense than the sagittal sinus, a grade 3 lesion was equal in intensity to the sagittal sinus, and a grade 4 lesion was more intense than the sagittal sinus.

For CTT scans the position of the head was adjusted such that the scanning plane formed an angle of 20 deg with the orbitomeatal line. The standard technique included four scans, of two contiguous slices each, resulting in eight images. The thickness of each slice was 13 mm. The lowest slice extended from the orbit to the foramen magnum. In those cases in which the main emphasis was on the posterior fossa, the scan was taken at a more acute angle (25–30 deg), and the lowest two scans were done using a smaller collimator so that the thickness of the slice measured 8 mm. To study the orbits in selected cases, scans with narrow collimation were done along a plane parallel to the orbitomeatal line. If a lesion was suspected to have increased vascularity, the CTT scan was repeated after intravenous administration of contrast material (100 cc of meglumine diatrizoate containing 282 mg of iodine per cc injected over a 4-min period).

The CTT scans were interpreted with reference to abnormalities in attenuation characteristics of the cerebral tissue. The lesion was thus described as having a high, low, or a combination of high and low densities. The size of the lesion was classified as small, medium, or large as described for radionuclide imaging. When a scan was repeated after contrast injection, any increase in the attenuation characteristics was noted. The CTT scans were also evaluated for presence of midline shift and ventricular size. The lateral ventricles were classified as normal or showing slight, moderate, or marked enlargement. The third and fourth ventricles and the cerebral sulci were described as normal or enlarged.

Results. There were 76 patients in this group. Lesions were detected in 68 patients (89%) by CTT scanning and in 65 patients (86%) by the radionuclide study (Table 9-1). An analysis of cases that were missed on one or both studies is shown in Table 9-2. The two gliomas that were not detected by radionuclide imaging were low-grade astrocytomas, and the one glioma not detected by the CTT scan was a cerebellar gliocytoma. In four patients with metastatic tumors the lesions were not detected by the CTT scan. Three of these lesions were demonstrated by radionuclide imaging. One metastatic tumor of the cerebellum was detected by the CTT scan but not by radionuclide imaging.

Table 9-1 shows that five of the six suprasellar masses were demonstrated by the CTT scan while three of the six had normal radionuclide scans. Of the three intracranial vascular malformations, one that was detected by radionuclide imaging was not detected by CTT scanning. It was a dural arteriovenous fistula between the

**TABLE 9-1. Detection of Intracranial Mass Lesions
by CTT and Radionuclide Imaging**

Diagnosis	Number of patients	Abnormal CTT Scan	Abnormal radionuclide imaging
Glioma	21	20	19
Meningioma*	5	5	5
Metastasis	28	24	26
Subdural hematoma	4	4	4
Suprasellar mass	6	5	3
Simple cyst	5	5	3
Intracranial AVM	3	2	2
Miscellaneous†	4	3	3
Total	76	68 (89%)	65 (86%)

* Other than suprasellar.
† Includes one case each of Herpes encephalitis, vascular granuloma of cerebellopontine angle, hamartoma, and cerebritis.

**TABLE 9-2. Intracranial Mass Lesions Not Detected
by CTT or Radionuclide Imaging**

Diagnosis	Lesion missed by CTT only	Lesion missed by radionuclide imaging only	Lesion missed by both procedures
Glioma	1	2	0
Metastasis	3	1	1
Suprasellar mass	1	3	0
Cyst	0	2	0
Vascular malformation	1	1	0
Granuloma of CPA	0	0	1
Total	6 (8%)	9 (12%)	2 (3%)

branches of the external carotid artery and the dural sinuses. A thrombosed cerebral vascular malformation was seen on the CTT scan but was not detected by radionuclide imaging. All five simple cysts were readily recognized on CTT images. The three patients who had rapid sequence radionuclide imaging showed decreased activity at the site of the cyst. The five meningiomas and four subdural hematomas in this series were demonstrated by both CTT and radionuclide imaging. However, a 2-cm-diam meningioma of the cerebral convexity was not detected by CTT scanning before contrast enhancement. In one patient with a subdural hematoma, the lesion was seen on the CTT scan but it was thought to be intracerebral. Rapid sequence radionuclide imaging demonstrated inward displacement of the middle cerebral artery activity, and static imaging revealed increased activity along the convexity on the same side, suggesting a subdural hematoma. Three extracerebral lesions were included in this study. Two orbital masses (a pseudotumor and an extension of ethmoid carcinoma) were detected by both the CTT and the radionuclide studies. A vascular malformation of the subtemporal fossa was detected by rapid sequence study and was not detected on the CTT scan. Radionuclide imaging and CTT scanning both detected two cases of cerebral inflammation (Herpes encephalitis and cerebritis) and a hamartoma whereas neither procedure detected a vascular granuloma of the cerebellopontine angle.

Morphological features. *Size.* Fifty-six cases in which the lesions were visualized on both the CTT and radionuclide scans were analyzed (Table 9-3). Most metastases and gliomas appeared larger

TABLE 9-3. Comparison of Size of Intracranial Mass Lesions Detected by Both CTT and Radionuclide Imaging

Diagnosis	Lesion same size on both studies	Lesion larger on CTT*	Total
Metastasis	4	19	23
Glioma	6	12	18
Meningioma	5	0	5
Subdural hematoma	4	0	4
Suprasellar lesion	2	0	2
Cyst	3	0	3
Vascular malformation	1	0	1
Total	25	31	56

* There were no lesions larger on radionuclide images than on CTT scans.

on the CTT than on the radionuclide scan. This larger appearance on CTT images is probably related to the detection of peritumoral edema by this technique. On the other hand, meningiomas, subdural hematomas, and suprasellar masses showed comparable sizes on both studies. The three cysts shown on rapid sequence scans (all large) appeared to be the same size on the CTT scans.

Vascularity. CTT scans were obtained before and after injections of contrast material on 21 patients. The results are shown in Table 9-4. Increased visibility of the lesion was noted after injection of contrast material in 17 of 21 cases (81%). There were several patterns of enhancement. Total opacification of the lesion (Fig. 9-1) was noted in all menigiomas, four metastases, one glioblastoma, and two vascular malformations, resulting in better visibility of the lesion in contrast to surrounding brain or surrounding edema. The vascular

Diagnosis	Increased density	No change	Total
Metastasis	7	2	9
Meningioma	5	0	5
Glioblastoma	3	0	3
Vascular malformation	2	1	3
Cyst	0	1	1
Total	17	4	21

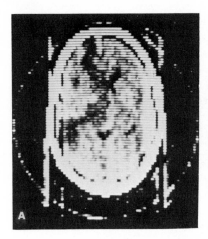 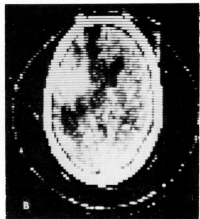

Fig. 9-1. Left sphenoid wing meningioma. (A) CTT scan before injection of contrast material. Ventricular system is displaced to right. Mass shows slightly increased density with surrounding lower density due to edema. (B) CTT scan after injection of contrast material. Tumor shows increase in density.

malformation that did not show contrast enhancement on the CTT scan was found at surgery to be a clotted arteriovenous malformation. In two cases, better visibility was associated with an apparent increase in the size of the lesion. A second pattern seen in one metastasis was visualization of the lesion that was originally detected only by surrounding edema. A third pattern seen in two metastases and two glioblastomas was the opacification of a rim surrounding a central cystic portion of the lesion (Fig. 9-2).

Rapid sequence radionuclide imaging was performed in 24 cases. Increased vascularity was demonstrated in all four meningiomas studied by this technique. In four of the five cases of glioblastoma the rapid sequence study was abnormal. In three of these, it showed increased vascularity associated with a large cystic component in the tumor. The rapid sequence imaging was abnormal in three cases of

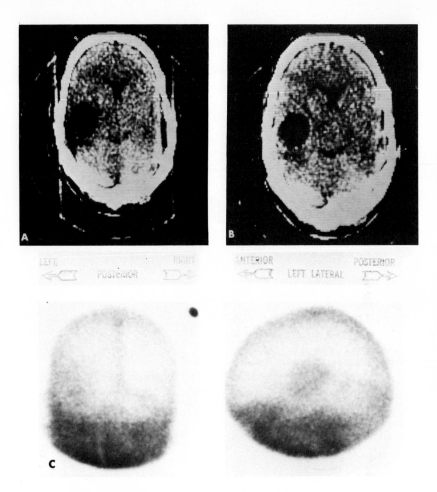

Fig. 9-2. Glioblastoma multiforme of left temporal lobe. (A) CTT scan before injection of contrast material shows cystic lesion with low density, similar to CSF density, in left temporal lobe. (B) CTT scan after contrast material shows cyst more well defined and outlined by rim of increased density. (C) Radionuclide brain images show large area of abnormal accumulation in left temporal region.

simple cysts, showing an area of decreased activity at the site of the lesion in each. The two cases of subdural hematoma studied by rapid sequence imaging showed decreased activity over the cerebral convexity in both (Fig. 9-3). Increased activity on rapid sequence images was seen in a suprasellar aneurysm but not in either of the two optic gliomas studied. The two vascular malformations showed increased activity on the rapid sequence study. One was a cerebral arteriovenous malformation and the other was a fistula between branches of the external carotid artery and the dural sinuses. Comparison between increased vascularity seen by CTT scanning with contrast material

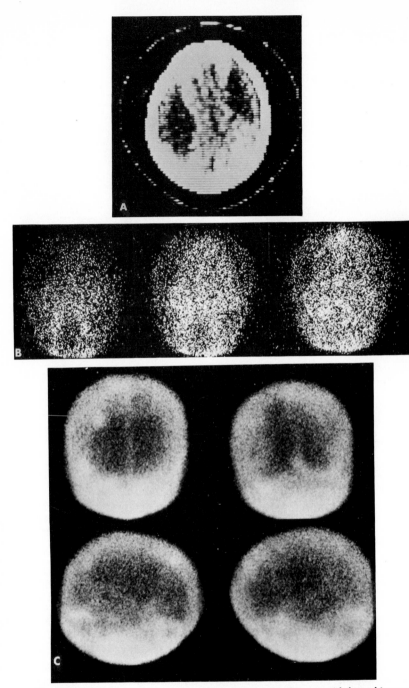

Fig. 9-3. Bilateral chronic subdural hematomas. (A) CTT scan with large biconvex regions of decreased density. (B) Rapid sequence radionuclide images demonstrate decreased activity over both cerebral convexities. (C) Static radionuclide images demonstrate increased activity over both convexities.

and increased activity on rapid sequence imaging in the same patient was possible in ten cases (Table 9-5). There was good correlation between the two procedures.

TABLE 9-5. Intracranial Mass Lesions: Comparison of Lesion Vascularity on CTT Scans and Rapid Sequence Radionuclide Images*

Diagnosis	CTT scan	Rapid sequence imaging
Meningioma	+	+
Meningioma	+	+
Meningioma	+	+
Metastasis	+	+
Metastasis	0	0
Metastasis	0	0
Cerebrovascular malformation	+	+
Durovascular malformation	0	+
Glioblastoma	+†	−‡
Glioblastoma	+	0

* +, Increased vascularity; 0, no evidence of increased vascularity.
† Increased vascularity in wall of cystic tumor.
‡ Decreased vascularity at site of cystic tumor.

Discussion. The overall detection rates of these lesions by CTT and radionuclide imaging are 89% and 86%, respectively. These figures are in agreement with previous reports concerning the accuracy of CTT scanning (1, 5) and radionuclide brain imaging (6-10). Although the difference between the detection rates is small, analysis of the cases with negative results by either or both techniques is of interest (Tables 9-1 and 9-2) and demonstrates the potential for complementary rather than competitive interaction of the two methods. Four of six neoplasms missed by CTT scanning were metastases while only one of six neoplasms missed by radionuclide scanning was a metastasis. Baker, et al (1) noted that the overall incidence of diagnostic errors for CTT scanning was 3.5%, while the error rate for metastases was 8.5%.

The likelihood of a negative result is also related to the site of the neoplasm. Three of six neoplasms not detected by CTT scans in our series were in the posterior fossa and one was in the suprasellar region. Conversely, among six neoplasms missed by the radionuclide study three were in the suprasellar region and one was in the posterior fossa. These observations suggest a higher relative accuracy for radionuclide imaging in posterior fossa lesions and for CTT scanning in suprasellar lesions. Radionuclide imaging is reported to detect only approximately 50% of suprasellar lesions (9, 11) and greater than 80% of posterior fossa mass lesions (12). Paxton and Ambrose (5) found that CTT demonstrated the lesion in 24 of 29 posterior fossa neoplasms.

CTT scanning offers an excellent method for determining the size and shape of the cerebral ventricles and other cerebrospinal fluid spaces, such as detecting porencephaly or cyst formation in a primary cerebral neoplasm (2, 4, 5). Radionuclide brain imaging is much less likely to detect cystic lesions or hydrocephalus since most brain lesions are detected by virtue of their increased activity relative to the normally low activity in the cerebral hemispheres. The accuracy of ^{99m}Tc brain imaging in detecting these lesions may be increased by the use of rapid sequence scintigraphy (13-16) in which the lesions appear as areas of decreased cerebral vascularity. The results of our study demonstrate the superiority of CTT scanning for detecting cystic lesions and hydrocephalus. However, the results also indicate that the sensitivity of radionuclide brain imaging for these hypovascular lesions is increased when a rapid sequence study is performed.

Lesions of the superficial convexity may occasionally be difficult to detect by CTT scanning. Subdural hematomas may not be detected because of their superficial location and their density characteristics (2-5). Acute subdural hematomas containing clotted blood are well visualized by transaxial tomography. Later, as clotted material undergoes changes the area develops a density similar to surrounding brain. If the ventricular system is not deformed in these cases, the transaxial tomograph may appear normal. The fluid of a chronic subdural hematoma may appear as a peripheral area of decreased density (Fig. 9-3). Radionuclide brain imaging in cases of suspected subdural hematoma has met with variable success. In adults 80–90% of chronic subdural hematomas can be detected by radionuclide imaging, especially if the lesion is more than 10 days old (17, 18). The diagnostic accuracy of the study in subdural collections can be improved by performing a rapid sequence study at the time of injection. A lack of perfusion in the peripheral convexity often occurs with subdural collections, and helps increase the sensitivity of the technique (19). In our study, four subdural hematomas were detected by both CTT and radionuclide imaging. However, the level of confidence in the results was greater with the radionuclide study in two of the cases.

Radionuclide imaging is a highly accurate method for detecting the presence of an arteriovenous malformation, especially when rapid sequence scintigraphy is employed (20). The irregular shape of the lesion and characteristic pattern of early increased activity and rapid washout on the rapid sequence study allows a reasonably specific diagnosis. Without the use of contrast enhancement, arteriovenous malformations may be difficult to delineate by CTT scanning. Because of the large venous blood pool, the lesion may be visualized as an area of low density (2). In other instances, the presence of a hematoma or calcification in the lesion may allow its detection (5). After the intravenous injection of an iodinated contrast material, the lesion becomes readily visible because of its high content of blood-borne contrast material (2) (Fig. 9-4). Our results indicate that the

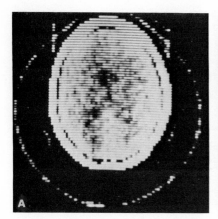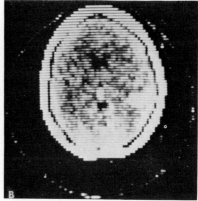

Fig. 9-4. Right parietal arteriovenous malformation. (A) CTT scan before image contrast enhancement. No abnormality is seen. (B) CTT scan after contrast enhancement by narrowing of window demonstrates lesion as increased density in right parietal region.

ability of CTT scanning to detect cerebrovascular malformations is comparable to radionuclide studies if contrast is used. However, it is of interest that in our series there were two vascular malformations fed exclusively by the external carotid artery. One drained into the dural sinuses and the other was totally extracerebral in the subtemporal region. Neither was shown on the CTT scan while both were well demonstrated on rapid sequence radionuclide imaging. Furthermore, it may be argued that a CTT study with contrast material is a more invasive procedure and exposes the patient to the adverse reactions associated with iodinated contrast material.

Computerized tomography and radionuclide imaging both have a high yield of positive results in intracranial mass lesions. Our results suggest a complementary role for the two procedures in the detection of cerebral mass lessions. At this time we are unable to determine which procedure should be used for initial examination in patients with a suspected mass lesion. CTT scanning provides better anatomical detail; however, a normal CTT scan does not exclude certain lesions that may be detected by radionuclide imaging. The CTT scan is better for detecting cystic lesions whereas radionuclide brain imaging is better for detecting metastatic lesions. Lesions in the suprasellar region are detected more frequently with CTT than with radionuclide brain imaging, but lesions in the superficial convexity and posterior fossa are more frequently detected with radionuclide imaging.

Cerebrovascular Disease

Methods. There were 29 patients with a final diagnosis of cerebrovascular accident, including 22 patients with recent infarction, 5 with intracerebral hemorrhage, and 2 with cerebral infarction occurring about 1 year prior to examination. The interval between the onset of symptoms and diagnostic imaging in this group of patients is shown in Table 9-6. In this study there was an inadvertent selection of patients

TABLE 9-6. Time Interval Between Cerebrovascular Accident and Imaging Studies

	0–2 days	2–7 days	More than 7 days
CTT scan	10	8	11
Radionuclide scan	12	8	9

resulting in an artificial bias. During the greater part of the period covered in this study there was only a single CTT unit in operation at our institute. As a result of the inevitable waiting list, patients with a negative radionuclide study were not studied by CTT scanning. It remains possible, therefore, that a group of patients with negative radionuclide studies and positive CTT scans was inadvertently omitted from the study. This will be discussed later.

Results. Among the 22 patients with recent infarction, 11 patients (50%) showed abnormality on the CTT scan and 19 (86%) showed abnormality on the radionuclide brain imaging (Table 9-7). The abnormalities on CTT scans consisted of decreased density of the brain tissue (Fig. 9-5). None of the patients had evidence of brain swelling on CTT scans. Nineteen of the patients showed abnormal accumulation on radionuclide imaging. Rapid sequence scintigraphy was done in 14 of these patients and showed early decreased vascularity in the involved hemisphere in 4 and was normal in 10. In addition to these 19 cases, there was one patient in whom the only abnormality of the radionuclide study was decreased vascularity on the rapid sequence study with no evidence of increased uptake on the delayed scan. This patient had a positive CTT scan. There were two patients in whom the CTT and radionuclide study were negative. Rapid sequence scintigraphy was done on one of these and it was also normal.

TABLE 9-7. Cerebrovascular Accidents: Results of Radionuclide and CTT Imaging

Diagnosis	Number of cases	Abnormal CTT scan	Abnormal Radionuclide imaging
Recent cerebral infarction	22	11 (50%)	19 (86%)
Recent intracerebral hematoma	5	5 (100%)	2 (40%)
Remote cerebral infarction	2	2 (100%)	1* (50%)

* Abnormal rapid sequence imaging and normal static image.

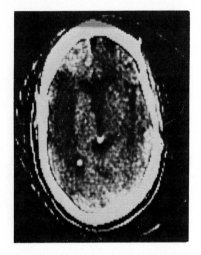

Fig. 9-5. Cerebral infarction. Lesion is shown as large area of decreased density in distribution of left middle cerebral artery.

In the 11 patients in whom a lesion was shown on CTT scan, a comparison was made of the size of the lesion on the CTT and radionuclide scans. In seven of these, the size of the lesion corresponded well on both studies. These were five medium-sized lesions, one small lesion, and one large lesion. There were three patients in whom the radionuclide scan showed a small lesion while the CTT scan showed medium-sized lesions in two and a large lesion in one. The remaining patient on whom the CTT study was positive showed a small lesion on the CTT scan and no abnormal uptake on radionuclide scan. However, the rapid sequence study in this patient showed decreased vascularity on the appropriate side in the territory of the middle cerebral artery. There were eight patients on whom the CTT scan was normal while radionuclide imaging showed increase uptake. Six of these showed a small lesion and two showed a medium-sized lesion.

The results of radionuclide and CTT studies were analyzed in relation to the time interval between the scan and the onset of symptoms in the 22 patients with cerebral infarction (Table 9-8). The

TABLE 9-8. Relationship of Findings of Radionuclide and CTT Studies to Time Interval after Onset of Cerebral Infarction

Time interval (days)	Number of cases	Abnormal scans	Abnormal studies (%)
Radionuclide imaging	22	19	86
0–7	13	11	85
7–21	6	5	83
>21	3	3	100
CTT scans	22	11	50
0–7	12	6	50
7–21	6	4	67
>21	4	1	25

studies were divided into three groups in which the time intervals were 0–7 days, 7–21 days, and greater than 21 days. The time interval between radionuclide and CTT studies ranged from 0 to 7 days in 21 cases. In one case it was 10 days. In 20 patients both the radionuclide and CTT studies were in the same group. There was one patient on whom the radionuclide study was in the first group (0–7 days) and the CTT was in the second group (7–21 days) with an interval of 5 days between the two studies. In the remaining patient, on whom the two scans were done 10 days apart, the radionuclide study was in the second group (7–21 days) and the CTT study in the third group (greater than 21 days). Table 9-8 demonstrates that there was little difference in the incidence of positive results between the three groups. The CTT studies showed a slight increase in the percentage of positive results in the interval 7–21 days after the episode (67%) and a lower incidence in the interval greater than 21 days (25%) than in the interval 0–7 days (50%). Unlike thromboembolic cerebral infarction, the intracerebral hematomas were detected by CTT scanning in all five patients included in this series (Table 9-7). The nature of the lesion was also determined, as distinct from infarction, in all five cases. In this group, radionuclide studies showed increased uptake indistinct from infarction in two patients. The remaining three patients showed normal radionuclide studies.

Discussion. The changes shown on CTT scans in patients with infarction have been described by New, et al (*3*) and Paxton and Ambrose (*5*). Both reports point to a series of changes based on the natural history of cerebral infarction. CTT scans obtained in the first few days after the ictus show a diffuse low density area involving the cortex and white matter with little or no midline displacement. Studies done more than 10 days after the initial episode show a more clearly defined density area. After 1 month or more, some patients show a well-defined cystic area with CSF density. New, et al (*3*) ascribe the early changes, within hours or days after the onset of infarction, to accompanying cerebral edema. He suggests that necrosis and phagocytosis result in the appearance, 10 days later, of a more well-defined margin and lower density of the lesion as compared to the edema of the earlier stage. If the area of necrosis is small, the lesion may become difficult to detect. When it is large, a remaining cavity with CSF density is seen at the site of an old infarct. The incidence of abnormal findings by CTT scanning in patients with cerebral infarction was reported to be 48% by Baker, et al (*1*) and 49% by Paxton and Ambrose (*5*). Our results are comparable (50%). None of our studies showed evidence of deformity of the ventricular system due to cerebral swelling. Davis and Pressman (*2*) also found that the majority of patients with cerebral infarction showed no such swelling.

The frequency of abnormal radionuclide studies in patients with cerebral infarction studied during the first week after the onset of symptoms (*21–27*) has been reported to vary between 20% and 40%. Welch, et al (*28*) in a study of 169 brain scans in patients with thromboembolic cerebral infarction reported 30% positive studies during the first week after the ictus and 52% positive findings in studies done greater than 10 days after the ictus. They also indicate a 27% incidence of abnormal studies in the first 2 days after the episode. In our study, the incidence of abnormal radionuclide scans in cerebral infarction was 86%. However, as indicated earlier there was an inadvertent selection of these patients related to the lack of availability of CTT scanning in the earlier months covered by this study. Therefore, we will not draw any conclusions from these figures regarding the relative accuracies of the two techniques in detecting infarcts.

Previous reports have demonstrated the efficacy of CTT scanning in detecting intracerebral hematomas (*3–5*). The high x-ray attenuation characteristic of clotted blood enables CTT scanning to accurately identify 100% (*4*) of intracerebral hematomas. Our results in this small series and our experience are in agreement with these findings. Moreover, we have studied three patients with intracerebral hematoma (one of them not included in this series) in whom the clinical diagnosis was one of thromboembolic infarction. It was only after CTT scanning that the nature of the lesion was determined.

The results of brain scans in patients with intracerebral hematoma in previous reports (*21, 25, 28–31*) show a wide range of incidence of abnormal scans (10–60%). In our experience (*28*) abnormal scans were seen in 43% of patients with intracerebral hematoma. The results in this study are in agreement with these previous results.

Cerebral Atrophy and Communicating Hydrocephalus

Radionuclide cisternography has been widely used in the evaluation of demented patients with suspected hydrocephalus (*32*) to demonstrate cerebrospinal fluid (CSF) flow patterns. Various cisternographic patterns have been described and correlated with the results of neurosurgical shunting (*32–36*). The pattern of communicating hydrocephalus in which there is ventricular reflux and stasis with subarachnoid block has been the one most frequently associated with an improvement in the patient's mentation after shunting (*33, 34*). Patients with cerebral atrophy having either normal studies or showing only slow flow of the radiopharmaceutical to the parasagittal region generally do not respond to shunting (*37*). Since the development of CTT scanning, its value in visualizing the ventricular system and the sulci over the convexities has been recognized. In most of the early reports, there were favorable statements about the prospects of the technique in respect to evaluation of hydrocephalus and cerebral atrophy (*32, 34*). However, no attempt was made in these studies to compare the results of CTT scanning with cisternography in the same way as cisternography has been compared with pneumoencephalography and CSF infusion. The purpose of this study was to compare the CTT and cisternographic patterns of the CSF pathways.

Methods. There were 44 patients with dementia included in this series. CTT studies and radionuclide cisternograms were done on all. Cisternography was performed following the lumbar intrathecal injection of 250–500 μCi of ^{111}In-DTPA. Multiple images of the head were obtained at approximately 4, 24, 48, and frequently 72 hr after injection. The images were evaluated for the presence and duration of ventricular reflux of the radiopharmaceutical and categorized in the following manner: no ventricular reflux; ventricular reflux persisting for less than 24 hr or for only 24 hr with subsequent clearance; or ventricular reflux lasting for 48 hr or longer. Convexity flow was classified as normal (parasagittal activity by 24 hr), slow (parasagittal region reached later than 24 hr), or block (parasagittal region not reached with no progression of tracer beyond the level of the block).

The images demonstrating the radiopharmaceutical patterns of ventricular reflux and stasis with a subarachnoid block were interpreted as communicating hydrocephalus of the obstructive type. The pattern demonstrating slow flow over the convexity with or without transient ventricular reflux was interpreted as cerebral atrophy. Intermediate patterns consisted of convexity block without ventricular reflux or with ventricular reflux but no stasis (32, 34).

CTT scans were done using an EMI scanner with the standard technique of obtaining eight images as described above. The size of the lateral ventricles and the cerebral sulci was evaluated on the CTT images. Lateral ventricular enlargement was graded as 1+ to 3+ corresponding to the subjective impression of the reader interpreting the enlargement as mild, moderate, or severe, respectively. Asymmetry of ventricular size was noted. Dilatation of the third ventricle, fourth ventricle, and cerebral sulci was noted as present or absent.

Results. The interpretations of the 44 cisternograms were as follows: cerebral atrophy (21), communicating hydrocephalus (12), intermediate pattern (9), and normal pattern (2). The findings are summarized in Table 9-9. CTT scans showed dilatation of the lateral

TABLE 9-9. CTT Scan Findings Compared with Cisternographic Patterns

	Cisternographic pattern		
	Communicating hydrocephalus	Atrophy	Intermediate
CTT scan findings	Number of patients (%)	Number of patients (%)	Number of patients (%)
Lateral ventricles	12	21	9
Severely enlarged	6 (50)	1 (5)	2 (22)
Moderately enlarged	6 (50)	11 (52)	3 (33)
Slightly enlarged	0 (0)	7 (33)	2 (22)
Not enlarged	0 (0)	2 (10)	2 (22)
Third ventricle	12	19	8
Enlarged	10 (83)	5 (26)	1 (12)
Not enlarged	2 (17)	14 (74)	7 (88)
Fourth ventricle	7	9	3
Enlarged	5 (71)	0 (0)	0 (0)
Not enlarged	2 (29)	9 (100)	3 (100)
Cerebral sulci	10	20	9
Enlarged	1 (10)	10 (50)	2 (22)
Not enlarged	9 (90)	10 (50)	7 (78)

ventricles in all 12 patients who had a cisternographic pattern of communicating hydrocephalus (Fig. 9-6). The ventricular dilatation was moderate in six and severe in six. Among the 21 patients with cisternograms interpreted as cerebral atrophy, the CTT scan showed different distributions of ventricular dilatation (Fig. 9-7). While in 11 patients the ventricles were moderately dilated, 7 patients showed only slight ventricular dilatation, and in 2 patients the lateral ventricles were normal. Severe dilatation was seen in only one of these 21

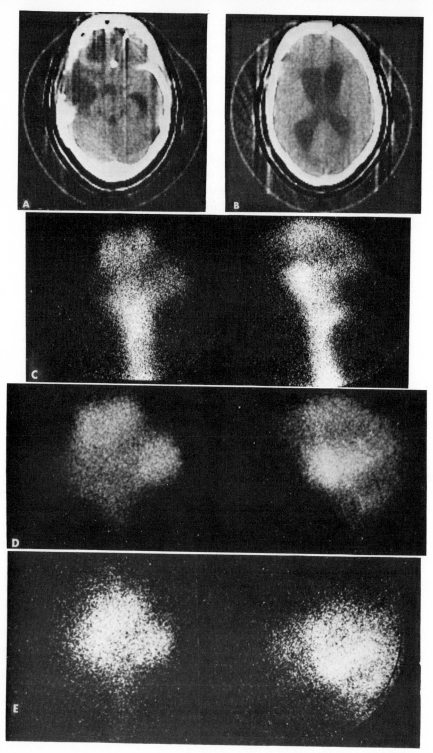

patients. Dilatation of the third ventricle was also more frequent in the group with the cisternographic pattern of communicating hydrocephalus (10 of 12 patients) than in the group with the pattern of atrophy (5 of 19). The fourth ventricle when visualized showed a more significant difference between the two groups. While none of the nine patients with the cisternographic pattern of atrophy and in whom the fourth ventricle was visualized showed dilatation of that ventricle, dilatation was present in five of seven patients in the group with the cisternographic pattern of communicating hydrocephalus. The cerebral sulci were visualized in the vast majority of the patients in both groups. Dilatation of the cerebral sulci was seen in half of the patients in the group with the cisternographic pattern of cerebral atrophy (Fig. 9-7). A low percentage (10%) of the communicating hydrocephalus group showed prominence of the sulci.

The group with an intermediate cisternographic pattern consisted of only nine patients. The size of the lateral ventricles varied from normal to severely dilated with no preponderance of a certain appearance. The third and fourth ventricles and the cerebral sulci were normal in most of these patients.

Discussion. Radionuclide cisternography is a reliable indicator of CSF flow patterns and has multiple applications including evaluation of patients with suspected hydrocephalus, CSF rhinnorhea, and CSF shunt function. Since the initial description of dementia and normal pressure hydrocephalus correctable by a CSF shunting procedure (*38*), many different procedures have been evaluated and correlated with the results of shunting. Even with a number of cisternographic and pneumoencephalographic criteria used, the results of shunting have often been disappointing. Patients demonstrating the cisternographic pattern of communicating hydrocephalus more frequently have a favorable response to shunting than those demonstrating the pattern of cerebral atrophy (*39*). However, some patients with the cisternographic pattern of atrophy and histological Alzheimer's disease have been reported to respond to shunting procedures (*40*).

Since some patients with dementia have a shunt-correctable process and since the radionuclide cisternogram has not always been a reliable predictor of patients who will respond to shunting, other procedures have been evaluated in patients with dementia. However, none seem to be definitive in separating patients into those with cerebral atrophy and those with communicating hydrocephalus. The pneumoencephalographic criteria (*40*) used for classifying a patient as

Fig. 9-6. (opposite page) Communicating hydrocephalus and left temporal porencephalic cyst. (A and B) CTT scans show symmetrical dilatation of lateral ventricles and cystic area with decreased density in left temporal region. (C, D, and E) Anterior and left lateral cisternographic images obtained at 4, 24, and 48 hr demonstrate ventricular reflux with stasis, an incisural block on right, and pooling of activity in left temporal area with no flow above that level.

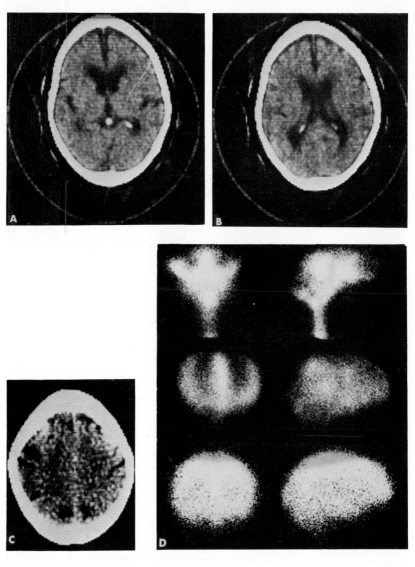

Fig. 9-7. Cerebral atrophy. (A, B, and C) CTT scans show dilatation of lateral ventricles and prominence of sulci. (D) Anterior and right lateral cisternographic images obtained at 4 hr (top), 24 hr (middle), and 48 hr (bottom) show transient ventricular reflux and slow flow over convexities.

having typical communicating hydrocephalus include a callosal angle of less than 120 deg, all four ventricles showing diffuse dilatation, and the basal cisterns being distended with air while no air appears in the subarachnoid space above the tentorial hiatus in spite of attempts to maneuver air in that direction. Other criteria in less typical cases include third ventricular width of 15 mm or more, supratentorial subarachnoid air limited to the space over the insulae and subfrontal region, or in the interhemisphere fissure, and normal width of the sulci. The pneumoencephalographic criteria of cerebral atrophy include widened sulci filled with air over the convexities of both frontal and parietal lobes. If the sulci were only partially filled, atrophy is diagnosed when only one of the less typical criteria of communicating hydrocephalus is present.

Several of the pneumoencephalographic criteria can be applied to the CTT scan. Although "filling" of the sulci cannot be evaluated by CTT scanning, their size can be demonstrated. In fact, absence of air over the hemispheres is of limited value in the diagnosis of communicating hydrocephalus. Air studies occasionally fail to demonstrate any peripheral cerebral sulci in patients with normal-sized ventricles and even in patients with cerebral atrophy.

We have developed a score chart for interpretating CTT scans relative to patients with dementia (Table 9-10). The total score is the

TABLE 9-10. CTT Scan Scoring for Patients with Dementia

CTT scan finding	Score
Lateral ventricles	
Normal	0
Slightly dilated	+1
Moderately dilated	+2
Severely dilated	+3
Third ventricle	
Normal	0
Dilated	+1
Fourth ventricle	
Normal	0
Dilated	+2
Cerebral sulci	
Normal	0
Dilated	−2

algebraic sum of the values given to each of the CTT findings. A dilated fourth ventricle scores higher than a dilated third ventricle. The total score (the algebraic sum of the four given values) is then interpreted as follows: a total score of 1 or less is interpreted as normal or cerebral atrophy; a total score of 3 or more is interpreted as communicating hydrocephalus; a score of 2 is considered an intermediate pattern.

We have applied this score system to the 44 CTT scans on patients who had cisternograms and we found a good correlation with the final diagnosis (Table 9-11). There were four patients on whom the CTT scan demonstrated normal ventricles and normal sulci. On two of them, an intermediate pattern was seen on cisternography. The

TABLE 9-11. Correlation between CTT Scans and
Cisternographic Patterns in Patients
with Dementia

Cisternographic pattern	CTT scan pattern				
	Communicating hydrocephalus	Atrophy	Intermediate	Normal	Total
Communicating hydrocephalus	10	0	2	0	12
Atrophy	1	15	4	1	21
Intermediate	2	2	3	2	9
Normal	0	1	0	1	2
Total	13	18	9	4	44

negative result of CTT scanning in these two patients was helpful and it was felt that there was no need for further evaluation of the patient on the basis of the cisternographic result.

A pattern of hydrocephalus on CTT scans cannot be described as "communicating" unless fourth ventricular dilatation and no evidence of a mass at its outlet are shown. The fourth ventricle was visualized in 7 out of 12 patients with the pattern of hydrocephalus. In only five of these patients was the fourth ventricle dilated and the diagnosis of communicating hydrocephalus made. Ventricular reflux was noted in 100% of cisternograms with the pattern of communicating hydrocephalus. The presence of ventricular reflux is evidence that the hydrocephalus is communicating with the subarachnoid space.

From these results, the complementary role of CTT scanning and cisternography can be seen. Moreover, in spite of the agreement between the CTT scan and cisternographic diagnosis in a high percentage of cases, CTT scanning does not provide the physiological dynamic information offered by the cisternogram. This includes ventricular reflux and site of block. Both are important in evaluating this ill-understood disease entity. Therefore, although we agree with the previous reports (3) that CTT is expected to replace pneumoencephalography in evaluating this disease, we disagree with the opinion that cisternography will have a diminished place in this respect.

Conclusions

CTT and radionuclide imaging are two noninvasive procedures that have a high rate of detection of intracranial masses and vascular malformations. Our results suggest a complementary role of both procedures. CTT scanning is superior for depicting anatomical detail and demonstrating cystic lesions and suprasellar masses. Radionuclide imaging is superior for detecting metastatic lesions and possibly masses in the superficial convexity or posterior fossa.

In cerebral thromboembolism, the results of both techniques may be comparable. Our data are not conclusive concerning this point. In patients with intracerebral hemorrhage, CTT scanning provides diagnostic information unobtainable by other techniques.

The results of CTT scanning and cisternography show a good correlation in patients being evaluated for communicating hydrocephalus or cerebral atrophy. We feel that CTT scanning has replaced pneumoencephalography in the evaluation of patients with dementia. Cisternography remains the procedure for providing dynamic information in this group of patients. In addition, complementary roles of CTT scanning and cisternography have been demonstrated.

Acknowledgment

The authors thank Barry A. Siegel and Ronald G. Evens for their help in preparing this manuscript and Michael Phelps, Carol Archer, and Tony Merlis for helpful discussions.

References

1. BAKER HL, CAMPBELL JK, HOUSER DW, et al: Computer assisted tomography of the head. An early evaluation. *Mayo Clin Proc* 49: 17–22, 1974

2. DAVIS DO, PRESSMAN BD: Computerized tomography of the brain. *Radiol Clin North Am* 12: 297–313, 1974

3. NEW PFJ, SCOTT WR, SCHNUR JA, et al: Computerized axial tomography with the EMI scanner. *Radiology* 110: 109–123, 1974

4. GAWLER J, BULL JWD, DuBOULAY GH, et al: Computer assisted tomography. Its place in investigation of suspected intracranial tumors. *Lancet* 2: 419–432, 1974

5. PAXTON R, AMBROSE J: The EMI scanner. A brief review of the first 650 patients. *Br J Radiol* 47: 530–565, 1974

6. HARPER PV, BECK R, CHARLESTON D, et al: Optimization of a scanning method using Tc-99m. *Nucleonics* 22: 50–54, 1964

7. WAGNER HN, HOLMES RA: The nervous system. In *Principles of Nuclear Medicine*, Wagner HN, ed, Philadelphia, WB Saunders, 1968, pp 655–689

8. O'MARA RE, MOZLEY JM: Current status of brain scanning. *Semin Nucl Med* 1: 7–31, 1971

9. SCHALL GL, QUINN JL III: Brain scanning. In *Nuclear Medicine*, Blahd WH, ed, New York, McGraw-Hill, 1971, pp 252–262

10. HANDA J: *Dynamic Aspects of Brain Scanning*, Baltimore, University Park Press, 1971, pp 80–82

11. EVENS RG, JAMES AE, ADATEPE MH: Brain scans in pituitary tumors. *Neurology* 21: 806–809, 1971

12. OSTERTAG C, MUNDINGER F, McDONNELL D, et al: Detection of 247 midline and posterior fossa tumors by combined scintigraphic and digital gammaencephalography. *J Neurosurg* 39: 224–229, 1974

13. MISHKIN F, TRUSKA J: The diagnosis of intracranial cysts by means of the brain scan. *Radiology* 90: 740–746, 1968

14. WEINBERG PE, FLOM RA: Intracranial subarachnoid cysts. *Radiology* 106: 329–333, 1973

15. CONWAY JJ, YARZUGARAY L, WELCH D: Radionuclide evaluation of the Dandy-Walker malformation and congenital arachnoid cyst of the posterior fossa. *Am J Roentgenol Radium Ther Nucl Med* 112: 306–314, 1971

16. MISHKIN F: Brain scanning in children. *Semin Nucl Med* 2: 328–342, 1972

17. ZINGESSER LH: Scanning in disease of the subdural space. *Semin Nucl Med* 1: 41–47, 1971

18. CONWAY JJ: Radionuclide imaging of the central nervous system in children. *Radiol Clin North Am* 10: 291–312, 1972

19. HOPKINS GB, KRISTENSEN KAB: Rapid sequential scintiphotography in the radionuclide detection of subdural hematomas. *J Nucl Med* 14: 288–296, 1973

20. LANDMAN S, ROSS P: Radionuclides in the diagnosis of arteriovenous malformations of the brain. *Radiology* 108: 635–639, 1973

21. TOW RE, WAGNER HN, DELAND FH, et al: Brain scanning in cerebral vascular disease. *JAMA* 207: 105–108, 1969

22. GLASGOW JL, CURRIER RD, GOODRICH JK, et al: Brain scans at varied intervals following C.V.A. *J Nucl Med* 6: 902–916, 1965

23. MORRISON RT, AFIFI AK, VAN ALLEN MW, et al: Scintiencephalography for the detection and localization of non-neoplastic intracranial lesions. *J Nucl Med* 6: 7–15, 1965

24. BROWN A, ZINGESSER L, SCHEINBERG LC: Radioactive mercury-labeled chlormerodrin scans in cerebrovascular accidents. *Neurology* 17: 405–411, 1967

25. OECONOMOS D: Gammaencephalography in cerebral vascular accidents. *Prog Brain Res* 30: 201–209, 1968

26. MARSHALL J, POPHAM MG: Radioactive brain scanning in the management of cerebrovascular disease. *J Neurol Neurosurg Psychiatry* 33: 201–204, 1970

27. MOLINARI GF, PIRCHER F, HEYMAN A: Serial brain scanning using technetium 99m in patients with cerebral infarction. *Neurology* 17: 627–636, 1967

28. WELCH DW, COLEMAN RE, HARDIN WB, et al: Brain scanning in cerebral vascular disease. A reappraisal. *Stroke* 6: 136–141, 1975

29. SHARMA SM, QUINN JL: Brain scans in autopsy proved cases of intracerebral hemorrhage. *Arch Neurol* 28: 270–271, 1973

30. OJEMANN RG, ARANOW S, SWEET WH: Scanning with positron-emitting isotopes in cerebrovascular disease. *Acta Radiol [Diagn] (Stockh)* 5: 894–905, 1966

31. OVERTON MC, HAYNIE TP, SNODGRASS SR: Brain scans in non-neoplastic intracranial lesions. *JAMA* 191: 431–436, 1965

32. HARBERT JC: Radionuclide cisternography. *Semin Nucl Med* 1: 90–106, 1971

33. McCULLOUGH DC, HARBERT JC, DiCHIRO G, et al: Prognostic criteria for cerebrospinal fluid shunting from isotope cisternography in communicating hydrocephalus. *Neurology* 20: 594–598, 1970

34. JAMES AE, NEW PFJ, HEINZ ER, et al: A cisternographic classification of hydrocephalus. *Am J Roentgenol Radium Ther Nucl Med* 115: 39–49, 1972

35. STAAB EV, ALLEN JH, YOUNG AB, et al: ^{131}I-HSA cisternograms and pneumoencephalography in evaluation of hydrocephalus. In *Cisternography and Hydrocephalus. A Symposium,* Harbert JC, McCullough DC, Luessenhop AJ, et al, eds, Springfield, Ill, Charles C Thomas, 1972, pp 235–248

36. FLEMING JFR, SHEPPARD RH, TURNER VM: CSF scanning in the evaluation of hydrocephalus: A classical review of 100 patients. In *Cisternography and Hydrocephalus. A Symposium,* Harbert JC, McCullough DC, Luessenhop AJ, et al, eds, Springfield, Ill, Charles C Thomas, 1972, pp 261–284

37. COBLENTZ JM, MATTIS S, ZINGESSER LH, et al: Presenile dementia. Clinical aspects and evaluation of cerebrospinal fluid dynamics. *Arch Neurol* 29: 299–308, 1973

38. ADAMS RD, FISHER CM, HAKIN S, et al: Symptomatic occult hydrocephalus with "normal" cerebrospinal-fluid pressure: A treatable syndrome. *N Engl J Med* 273: 117–126, 1965

39. OJEMANN RG, FISHER CM, ADAMS RD, et al: Further experience with the syndrome of "normal pressure hydrocephalus." *J Neurosurg* 31: 279–297, 1969

40. LEMAY M, NEW PF: Pneumoencephalography and isotope cisternography in the diagnosis of occult normal pressure hydrocephalus. *Radiology* 96: 347–358, 1970

Chapter **10**

Clinical Comparison of Radionuclide Brain Imaging and Computerized Transmission Tomography, II

Anthony M. Passalaqua, Philip Braunstein,
Irvin I. Kricheff, Thomas P. Naidich,
and Norman E. Chase

T he recent introduction of computerized transaxial tomography (CTT) scanning has apparently added a new dimension to the diagnosis of neurological diseases. Since radionuclide brain scanning has long been established as a valuable diagnostic technique, it has become important to compare the relative values of these two noninvasive procedures. This comparative study of the two techniques was undertaken for this purpose.

Materials and Methods

Our study includes patients examined during the first 6 months of the operation of the EMI scanner at the New York University Medical Center. During this period 1,055 EMI scans (CTT) and 1,116 radionuclide brain scans were performed. From this group we selected 277 patients having both CTT and radionuclide scans performed within 30 days of one another. There was no neurosurgical treatment and no overt change in neurological findings in the interval between studies among these patients. Both studies were scheduled independently of one another and in the usual routine of the referring physician. No attempt was made to influence the clinician's choice of studies to be performed or to solicit cooperation in a combined study.

The technique for radionuclide scans included premedication with 400 mg of KClO$_4$ at least 30 min before administration of the radionuclide. A rapid sequence flow study was routinely obtained with an Anger camera immediately following intravenous injection of a 10-mCi bolus of ^{99m}Tc-pertechnetate. Static scans were performed with an Anger camera or rectilinear scanner at 1–3 hr following injection. Routine views included anterior, posterior, and lateral projections. A Towne's view was added in all Anger camera studies. Other views were occasionally obtained as appropriate. If the clinical history suggested the possibility of a subdural hematoma or metastasis, the static scans were delayed for at least 3 hr.

The CTT studies included three or four scans generating six to eight tomographic slices, each inclined at 20 deg to the orbitomeatal line. Results were displayed in an 80 × 80 matrix and Polaroid photographs were taken for the permanent record. Digital information was also printed out for reference and was available at the time of interpretation. Studies with contrast agents were performed selectively. During the first 3 months of the study, most patients were given 15 gm of iodine (50 cc of 60% renographin) and scanned 45 min after injection. Subsequently, patients were given 30 gm of iodine (100 cc of 60% renographin or 200 cc of 30% renographin) by rapid infusion and scanned immediately after injection.

Final clinical diagnosis in each patient was based on history, physical and neurological examinations, radionuclide scan, CTT scan, and other neuroradiological procedures as indicated. Clinical followup was included when available, and in some cases surgical or pathological confirmation was obtained.

Results

The distribution of the final diagnoses among the 277 patients is given in Table 10-1. We will present the results of each group separately.

Normal. Among the 119 patients with a final diagnosis of normal, three patients had CTT scans that were initially read as positive. Each of these had CTT scans repeated 4–6 months later that were interpreted as normal. Retrospective reviews of the three earlier studies were interpreted as normal in one case and equivocal in the other two cases. These false positives are now attributed to errors in interpretation resulting from inexperience. There were no false-positive radionuclide scans.

Primary tumors. There were 39 patients with primary brain

TABLE 10-1. Final Diagnoses of 277 Patients Studied
by CTT and Radionuclide Imaging

Normal	119
Cerebral atrophy	49
Primary brain tumor	39
Metastatic tumor	26
Cerebrovascular accident	34
Arteriovenous malformation	5
Subdural hematoma	1
Hydrocephalus	4
Total	277

tumors. Twenty-three of these patients had both scans performed within an interval of 3 days. In eight patients the interval was within 7 days, in four between 8 and 18 days, and in the remaining four between 20 and 27 days. All except one had cerebral angiography, and 20 had surgical biopsies. In 32 patients tumors were located within the cerebral hemispheres, and in 7 within the posterior fossa.

The distribution of the histological types is shown in Table 10-2.

TABLE 10-2. Primary Tumors

Tumor	Number	False negatives Radionuclide scan	CTT
Glioma	20	3	2
Meningioma	7	0	0
Pituitary adenoma	3	1	0
Craniopharyngioma	1	1	0
Acoustic neuroma	1	0	1
Miscellaneous	7	4	1
Total	39	9	4

The miscellaneous category included tumors of the following types: pinealoma, colloid cyst of the third ventricle, choroid plexus papilloma of the fourth ventricle, neuroma of the fifth nerve, fourth ventricular cholesteatoma, hamartoma, and an uncategorized malignant tumor of the left cavernous sinus, believed to be a teratoma.

The false-negative radionuclide and CTT scans are enumerated in Table 10-2 and further categorized in Table 10-3. It can be seen that radionuclide scans detected 30 of 39 primary tumors (77%) and that CTT scans detected 35 of 39 (90%).

The patients with the falsely negative CTT scans who had a glioma of the brain stem involving the thalamus and the acoustic

TABLE 10-3. False-Negative Primary Tumors

Radionuclide scans	CTT
Glioma of brain stem	Glioma involving brain stem
Medulloblastoma of	and thalamus*
cerebellum	Recurrent anaplastic astrocytoma
Astrocytoma of left	of left cerebral hemisphere
cerebral hemisphere	Acoustic neuroma*
Pituitary adenoma	Uncategorized malignant tumor
Craniopharyngioma	of left cavernous sinus
Pinealoma	
Colloid cyst of third	
ventricle	
Cholesteatoma	
Neuroma of fifth nerve	

* Includes CTT scans repeated with contrast material.

neuroma had repeat scans with contrast media that were again falsely negative.

Further comparison of the relative sensitivities of the two methods is illustrated in Table 10-4. Both techniques were more

TABLE 10-4. Primary Tumors

Location	Positive/total	Sensitivity (%)
Cerebral hemispheres		
Radionuclide scans	26/32	81
CTT scans	30/32	94
Posterior fossa		
Radionuclide scans	4/7	57
CTT scans	5/7	71
Radionuclide scans, total	30/39	77
CTT scans, total	35/39	90
Combined results of both techniques	39/39	100

sensitive in detecting lesions in the cerebral hemispheres than in the posterior fossa. It is important to note that by performing both procedures on each of the patients in this group, every lesion (100%) was detected.

Metastatic tumors. There were 26 patients with metastatic disease to the brain. All except two had histologically proven primary tumors. One of these had a mass in the left lung on a chest radiograph that was thought to be a bronchogenic carcinoma. The second patient had an unknown primary and multiple metastatic lesions. All patients in this group had both procedures performed within 1 week of each other, except for one patient, in whom the radionuclide scan was done 17 days after the CTT scan. Both procedures were positive in this patient.

Multiple cerebral lesions were found in 16 patients by one or both methods. The radionuclide scans detected multiple lesions in 7 patients, while CTT scans revealed multiple lesions in 13.

The relative sensitivities of the two techniques are summarized in Table 10-5. Among the five patients with falsely negative radionuclide

TABLE 10-5. Metastatic Tumors

Location	Positive/total	Sensitivity (%)
Cerebral hemispheres		
Radionuclide scans	16/17	94
CTT scans	17/17	100
Posterior fossa		
Radionuclide scans	5/9	56
CTT scans	6/9	67
Combined results of both techniques	7/9	78
Radionuclide scans, total	21/26	81
CTT scans, total	23/26	88
Combined results of both techniques	24/26	92

scans, three had metastatic carcinoma of the lung, one had reticulum cell sarcoma with a primary in the breast, and one had a plasmacytoma. All three patients with falsely negative CTT scans had metastases in the posterior fossa. Two were from the lung and one from the breast. The two from the lung were also negative by radionuclide scan, but were positive on repeat CTT scans performed with contrast material. The metastatic lesion from the breast was positive by radionuclide scan. This patient did not have a repeat CTT scan with contrast material. As in the primary tumors, both techniques were more sensitive in detecting lesions in the cerebral hemispheres than in the posterior fossa, and the combined results of both were more sensitive than those of either alone in both regions.

Arteriovenous malformations. There were five patients with arteriovenous malformations, all proven by cerebral angiography. All five (100%) were clearly positive by the static radionuclide scans. Three rapid sequence flow studies were clearly positive, revealing localized rapid accumulation of activity with washout in the venous phases of the studies. Four patients had CTT scans without contrast. Two of the four were positive. One of these revealed speckled foci of increased absorption presumably caused by small calcifications within the malformation. Lesions were seen in both patients who had CTT scans after injection of contrast material. One of these lesions had been negative in the CTT scan performed without contrast agent, while the other lesion was not studied without the contrast agent.

Cerebrovascular accidents. There were 34 patients with cerebrovascular accidents. Twenty-seven had ischemic infarcts and seven had intraparenchymal hemorrhages. Fifteen patients had angiograms showing vascular occlusive disease, avascular masses, or aneurysms. In 12 patients, the radionuclide and CTT scans were performed on the same day. In seven patients, there was an interval of 2–3 days between the two studies; in nine patients, 4–5 days; in four patients, 6–9 days; in one patient, 18 days; and in one patient, 21 days.

As shown in Table 10-6, there were six false-negative radionuclide

TABLE 10-6. Cerebrovascular Accidents with False-Negative Radionuclide Scans

	Days between onset of symptoms and radionuclide scan	Days between radionuclide scan and CTT scan	Angiography
Cerebral infarct	30	2	None
Cerebral infarct	4	3	None
Cerebral infarct	?	4	+
Cerebral infarct	3,7	1	None
Brain stem infarct	9	4	None
Intracerebral hemorrhage	14	2	+

scans. These included four hemispheric infarctions, one infarction of the brain stem, and one intracerebral hemorrhage. The time between onset of clinical symptoms and performance of the scans ranged from 3 to 30 days. One patient had a repeat scan at 7 days, which was again negative.

There were also six false-negative CTT scans as shown in Table 10-7. All were cerebral infarcts. Three had cerebral angiograms with findings of cerebral infarction. The time between the onset of symptoms and the performance of CTT scans ranged from 2 to 60 days. One scan repeated at 17 days was again negative, and one scan repeated with contrast material was also negative.

The sensitivity of each method in the detection of cerebrovascular accidents was 82% (28 of 34 patients). However, the combination of both procedures detected all (100%) that were studied.

Cerebral atrophy and hydrocephalus. There were 53 patients with cerebral atrophy and hydrocephalus (Table 10-1). CTT scans were able to visualize the CSF spaces and were thus useful in the evaluation of

TABLE 10-7. Cerebrovascular Accidents with
False-Negative CTT Scans

	Days between onset of symptoms and CTT scan	Days between radionuclide scan and CTT scan	Angiography
Cerebral infarct	2,17	7	+
Cerebral infarct	60	1	+
Cerebral infarct	60	3	+
Cerebral infarct	10	5	None
Cerebral infarct	7	1	None
Cerebral infarct	14	0	None

these conditions. Radionuclide brain scanning is of little clinical value in detection of atrophy or hydrocephalus.

Subdural hematoma. The one subdural hematoma in this study, proven by angiography, was detected by the radionuclide scan but was negative by CTT scan.

Table 10-8 shows a comparison of the overall sensitivities of

TABLE 10-8. Radionuclide and CTT Scans (without Contrast Material): a Comparison of Overall Sensitivity

Method	Positive/total
Radionuclide scan	84/105 (80%)
CTT scan	88/105 (84%)
Combined radionuclide and CTT scans	103/105 (98%)

radionuclide and CTT scans in the five categories of patients in this study: those with primary tumor, metastasis, arteriovenous malformation, cerebrovascular accident, and subdural hematoma. These data include only CTT scans without contrast material. It is important to note that the combination of radionuclide scans and CTT scans without contrast detected 98% of these lesions, a percentage significantly higher than that of either procedure alone.

Discussion

Before drawing firm conclusions from this study, certain limitations should be emphasized. The number of cases, especially in some of the rarer categories, is so small that they can only point to a trend rather than provide statistically conclusive data. There is an ongoing national cooperative study to compare the efficacy of CTT and radionuclide brain scanning under more controlled and optimized conditions. It is also important to note that the evaluation of CTT scanning in this study covers an early period in which we were relatively inexperienced in interpretation and technique and were employing an 80 × 80 matrix instead of the 160 × 160 matrix now in use. Early studies were generally done without contrast material, while more recently it appears that as many as 50% of patients are receiving CTT scans both without and with contrast agents as an initial evaluation.

Nevertheless, it is clear even at this stage that CTT scanning is a remarkably effective new neurodiagnostic tool. In most categories, it may perform somewhat better than radionuclide scanning. Furthermore, it is useful in evaluating cerebral atrophy and hydrocephalus, in which radionuclide scanning is not as helpful. On the other hand, it appears that the anticipation that CTT scanning might be completely sensitive, accurate, and definitive is, not unexpectedly, unrealistic, although greater specificity has been claimed by some authors (1). It is becoming apparent that there are certain lesions that are more readily detected by CTT scanning (e.g., low-grade gliomas, lesions of the brain stem, and the multiplicity of metastatic lesions) while others are more effectively demonstrated by radionuclide scanning (e.g., arteriovenous malformations, meningiomas, and chronic subdural hematomas). Similar findings have been reported by others (2) although not all reports agree (3).

The impressive sensitivity of the combination of these two noninvasive techniques is striking, even in regions such as the posterior fossa and near the base of the skull where each alone leaves much to be desired. We feel that this impressive combined accuracy is probably the most significant finding in our study.

Apart from specific circumstances in which one procedure may be indicated over the other, the question of how widely each should be used will most certainly be influenced by economic considerations. Radionuclide scans utilizing widely available equipment will continue to be more readily available in the near future. Although CTT scanning may be the more accurate method in some circumstances, one may question whether this warrants the cost of making it available for all brain screening. Perhaps a more important consideration is the apparently increased sensitivity achieved by combining the two techniques. How does this affect the design of an ideal screening program? Should the less expensive or more readily available procedure be done first, and, if negative or if other information is still desired, should it be followed by the other technique? The widespread use of this combined approach may well decrease the number of cerebral angiograms and pneumoencephalograms. In our institution, it is now unusual for the clinician to request either of these procedures if the radionuclide and CTT scans are both negative.

The efficacy of performing CTT scanning both with and without contrast material is another point to consider. Although it is apparent that a CTT scan repeated with contrast material following a negative study will increase sensitivity for some lesions, in our experience the combination of radionuclide scanning and CTT scanning without contrast material detected 98% of lesions (excluding cerebral atrophy and hydrocephalus). This probably exceeds the sensitivity of the combined CTT studies and in our institution is about 30% less expensive. Furthermore, the injection of contrast material is not without risk. Witten, et al (4) reported a 5.1% incidence of mild reaction to contrast material, a 0.09% incidence of severe reaction to contrast material, and one death in nearly 33,000 individuals.

Conclusions

CTT scanning is a valuable new neurodiagnostic tool that appears to be generally more sensitive than radionuclide brain scanning. Both procedures will continue to be useful, their relative utilizations being based on clinical and economic factors. The combination of radionuclide and CTT imaging appears to be outstandingly effective, as well as less expensive and safer than the combination of CTT scans with and without contrast material.

References

1. BAKER HL, CAMPBELL JK, HOUSER DW, et al: Computer assisted tomography of the head: an early evaluation. *Mayo Clin Proc* 49: 17–27, 1974

2. DAVIS DO, PRESSMAN BD: Computerized tomography of the brain. *Radiol Clin North Am* 12: 297–312, 1974

3. NEW PFJ, SCOTT WR, SCHUR JA, et al: Computed tomography with the EMI scanner in the diagnosis of primary and metastatic intracranial neoplasms. *Radiology* 114: 75–87, 1975

4. WITTEN DM, FREDERICK DH, HIRSCH D, et al: Acute reactions to urographic contrast medium. *Am J Roentgenol Radium Ther Nucl Med* 199: 832–840, 1973

A Preliminary Comparison between ACTA Scans and Radionuclide Imaging Studies of the Central Nervous System

John C. Harbert, Stewart P. Axelbaum,
Dieter Schellinger, and Giovanni DiChiro

The ACTA scanner (Automatic Computerized Transverse Axial Scanner) is a new version of computer-assisted transaxial tomography designed and built at Georgetown University by Dr. Robert S. Ledley. This device has been described in detail elsewhere (*1*) and the mechanics will only be discussed briefly here.

Attenuation coefficients are determined for a transverse slice of the scanned object by translating an x-ray beam along a 24- or 48-cm-long path, rotating 1 deg, and repeating the scan through 180 deg. Two NaI(Tl) crystals move in tandem opposite the x-ray source detecting those photons transmitted through the object. On each scan pass, 160 discrete readings are measured and processed. The final matrix consists of 25,600 cells. The size of each cell depends on the pass length. The two adjacent sections obtained are 7.5-mm thick separated by 3 mm (center-to-center separation, 10.5 mm). By this means, large and small objects can be scanned with maximum resolution consistent with the size of the computer core. The algorithm for reconstructing the transverse section image is based on two-dimensional Fourier analysis (see Chapter 8).

Once the attenuation coefficients are determined, the two sections are displayed as television images either in color or in black and white with 16 colors or gray levels. The colors or gray levels correspond to the relative attenuation coefficients. The attenuation number may range in value from 0 to 2,048. On the display, the mean value and the range of display about the mean can be varied widely to produce an image of optimum contrast. The scan time requires 4½–5½ min depending on the length of the scan pass. The image is displayed immediately on completion of the scan. The absorbed radiation dose to the skin is at most 1.8 rads per scan with very little overlap between scanned areas.

The ACTA scanner uses a different algorithm and electronic processing than the EMI scanner and requires no water jacket interposed between the x-ray source and the part scanned. This unique feature allows the entire body to be scanned, thus extending the diagnostic applications considerably.

Preliminary reports on the range of pathological material scanned by the ACTA scanner have been published (2–4). During the first 8 months of operation, scanning time has been divided among clinical diagnostic studies, clinical research, and technical improvements. At this writing approximately 600 patients have been analyzed in detail. These include 528 cerebral studies and 72 extracerebral scans. We consider a detailed evaluation of the instrument's accuracy premature at this time. However, a number of comparisons can be made, particularly as they relate to radionuclide scanning.

Intracerebral Lesions

Table 11-1 lists 78 patients on whom both ACTA and radionuclide scans were performed. All had proven diagnoses of intracerebral lesions. The ACTA scans included seven cases in which the lesion was visualized only after intravenous administration of contrast agent and eight cases which were diagnosed by secondary manifestations, such as ventricular or choroid plexus shift rather than by visualization of the lesion itself. All radionuclide brain scans were performed using 15 mCi of ^{99m}Tc-pertechnetate. Rapid flow studies were recorded on 35-mm film with a Searle Radiographics HP scintillation camera. Static images were obtained 1.5–2.0 hr after injection with a dual-head Ohio-Nuclear scanner with 5-in.-diam detectors. Brain scans were interpreted as positive only if the scan abnormality corresponded to the proven anatomic lesion.

All seven patients in Table 11-1 with intracerebral hematomas had easily discernible, dense intracerebral lesions on ACTA scans. As others have reported (5, 6), computerized transaxial tomography is extremely sensitive for the detection and precise localization of even small intracerebral hematomas because of the high value of their

TABLE 11-1. Comparison of ACTA Scans and Radionuclide Scans in Proved Intracerebral Lesions

Disease process	No.	ACTA positive/ nuclide positive	ACTA positive/ nuclide negative	ACTA negative/ nuclide positive	ACTA negative/ nuclide negative
Intracerebral hematoma	7	3	4	0	0
Subdural hematoma	10	6	1	3	0
Arteriovenous malformation	4	2	1	1	0
Abscess	1	1	0	0	0
Acute infarction	10	2	1	4	3
Neoplasms (46)					
Astrocytoma	17	7	4	5	1
Oligodendroglioma	1	1	1	0	0
Medulloblastoma	2	1	0	1	0
Hemangioblastoma	1	0	0	1	0
Meningioma	7	5	0	2	0
Pituitary adenoma	2	0	0	1	1
Metastasis	13	9	0	3	0
Craniopharyngioma	1	1	0	0	1
Chloroma	1	0	0	1	0
Pinealoma	1	0	0	0	1
Total	78	38	12	22	7

x-ray attenuation coefficient. All four patients with negative radionuclide scans had basal ganglia hemorrhages, locations that are difficult to study for any type of pathology by radionuclide scanning (Fig. 11-1).

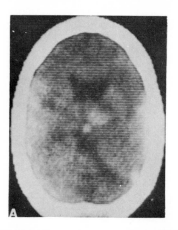

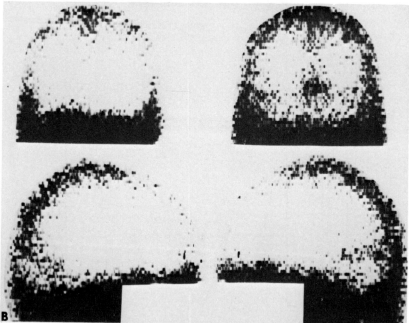

Fig. 11-1. ACTA and radionuclide scans of patient with hematoma. (A) ACTA scan shows dense hematoma in right thalamus with line of edema where clot encroaches on internal capsule. (B) Radionuclide scan is normal.

Radionuclide scans were somewhat more accurate in localizing subdural hematomas than ACTA scans; however, they were scarcely more specific. Four of the six studies positive by ACTA scan were found to have only a ventricular shift while the radionuclide scan demonstrated the typical crescent pattern of increased peripheral activity (Fig. 11-2). This crescent pattern can be caused by a variety

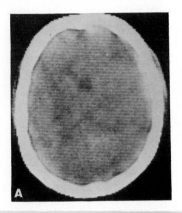

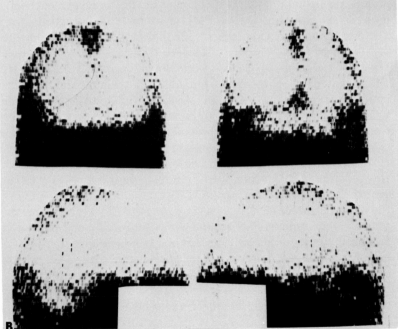

Fig. 11-2. ACTA and radionuclide scans of patient with subdural hematoma. (A) ACTA scan shows leftward shift of frontal horns. Dense zone outside right posterior frontal lobe is artifact. (B) Radionuclide scan demonstrates typical crescent pattern of peripheral activity.

of pathological processes including traumatic, inflammatory, and neoplastic lesions of the skull, scalp, and brain. A combination of radionuclide and ACTA scanning helps differentiate between the skull and scalp lesions, but may not distinguish between lesions such as peripheral brain tumor and subdural hematoma. Interpretation becomes especially difficult after previous surgery in which bone flaps and metal clips can project artifacts across the ACTA images. In these cases angiography will probably be required for specific diagnosis. The three patients with negative ACTA scans all had bilateral subdural hematomas without ventricular shift. Three other patients had normal ACTA scans and arteriograms but had suspected subdural hematomas by radionuclide scans. In these patients there were technical artifacts in the radionuclide scans caused by slight head rotation that probably could have been eliminated by studies repeated with a scintillation camera.

ACTA scanning and brain scanning were complementary in the detection of arteriovenous malformations, each technique missing one, but not in the same case. However, it should be noted that two of the three ACTA scan cases were positive by virtue of previous intracerebral bleeding. Paxton and Ambrose (5) have recently reported seeing intracerebral hematoma as the only evidence of arteriovenous malformation by EMI scans in 10 of 14 patients.

Among 46 proven neoplasms, 38 (83%) of the radionuclide scans were positive and 28 (61%) of the ACTA scans were positive. The negative radionuclide scans were found primarily among well-differentiated astrocytomas (2), brain-stem or thalamic gliomas (2), and brain-floor locations (4), all lesions or locations in which radionuclide scans are known to be less sensitive. Four tumors (9%) were missed by both scanning procedures. One pituitary adenoma did not extend out of the sella and was not included in this survey. However, another adenoma did extend beyond the sella and, while two separate ACTA scans were negative, the tumor was well demonstrated by the radionuclide scan.

Among intracranial mass lesions, the ACTA scanner was more sensitive than radionuclide scanning only for intracerebral hematoma, an unusually dense lesion. The accuracy of radionuclide brain scanning for all of the intracranial lesions studied was 77%, which is comparable to most reported series (7–9; Chapter 1).

The ACTA scans also demonstrated less accuracy for these same lesions (63%) than has been reported for the EMI scanner in four recent studies (5, 10–12). A number of reasons for this discrepancy are suggested by our analysis. The most crucial is patient motion. The EMI scanner has a water jacket and better patient restraint devices than the ACTA scanner. A new head-holding device is currently being designed that will provide better immobilization. Intrinsic resolution appears to be about equal for the ACTA and EMI scanners in phantom studies. However, there is one particular artifact that appears frequently on ACTA images but apparently not on EMI images, namely a bilateral density and frontoposterior lucency that we have termed "cupping and capping" (Fig. 11-3). These artifacts

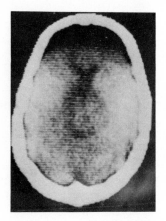

Fig. 11-3. Lateral (white) and frontal (dark) "cupping and capping" artifacts.

may obscure pathology in these areas. Work is currently being conducted to eliminate this problem. Also, at this stage of development we are unable to delineate the fine density differences found in some types of intracranial lesions. However, with the technical improvements already made and in progress, we feel confident that analysis of the next 600 cases will demonstrate much higher ACTA scan accuracy.

Hydrocephalus and Atrophy

Twenty adults were studied by radionuclide cisternography and ACTA scans (Table 11-2). Images were obtained with a scintillation camera at 1, 3, 6, 24, and 48 hr after intrathecal injection of ^{111}In-DTPA or ^{169}Yb-DTPA. All five adults with normal ventricular size had normal cisternographic patterns. Of five adults with atrophy, one patient had ventricular reflux and all had delayed clearance of the radiopharmaceutical (Fig. 11-4). Only two patients with ACTA scan findings of hydrocephalus without atrophy had no ventricular reflux. One of these had mild atrophy by pneumoencephalography that was unaccountably missed by ACTA scanning. The second patient has been lost to followup. The other eight hydrocephalics had a variety of cisternographic patterns, all abnormal.

A larger series than this is needed to establish firm criteria indicating the need for cisternography after computer-assisted tomographic scanning. It may be that cisternography will no longer be

ACTA scan diagnosis	Cisternographic pattern	Number	
		Adults	Children
Normal ventricular size	No ventricular reflux	5	1
Hydrocephalus and	No ventricular reflux	4	0
atrophy	Ventricular reflux	1	0
Hydrocephalus	No ventricular reflux	2	9
without atrophy	Ventricular reflux	8	4
Total		20	14

considered an initial test for normal-pressure hydrocephalus. ACTA scanning is so accurate in assessing ventricular size that without evidence of ventricular dilatation there may be little value to be gained by cisternography. These preliminary data suggest that ACTA scanning is relatively sensitive in detecting atrophy and these patients probably do not require cisternography. Thus of the 20 adults studied, only 8, all with unexplained hydrocephalus, received additional benefit from cisternography. In the future, one can anticipate that the best screening test for dementia will be computer-assisted tomography and cisternography and that radionuclide brain scanning will be reserved for those patients without atrophy and/or with hydrocephalus.

Fourteen children were evaluated by cisternography and ACTA scanning. Only one patient had normal ventricular size. He had a normal cisternogram and was felt to have asymptomatic macrocephaly. Nine patients had hydrocephalus without ventricular reflux. Four of these nine were found by contrast studies to have noncommunication and were shunted; five were felt to have arrested hydrocephalus and continued to be followed. One patient had a porencephalic cyst demonstrated by both studies (Fig. 11-5). Four children had significant ventricular reflux; three were shunted, and one with very mild clinical manifestations is being followed in hope of eventual compensation.

ACTA scanning has been very useful in following ventricular size in children both as followup and to judge the response to shunting. In patients with asymptomatic macrocephaly and only mildly dilated

Fig. 11-4. ACTA scans and cisternogram of patient with cerebral atrophy. (A) ACTA scan shows dilated ventricles and prominent intrahemispheric fissure. (B) ACTA scan at higher cut shows dilated cortical sulci. (C) Cisternograms demonstrate delayed ascent of [169]Yb-DTPA over convexities and no ventricular reflux.

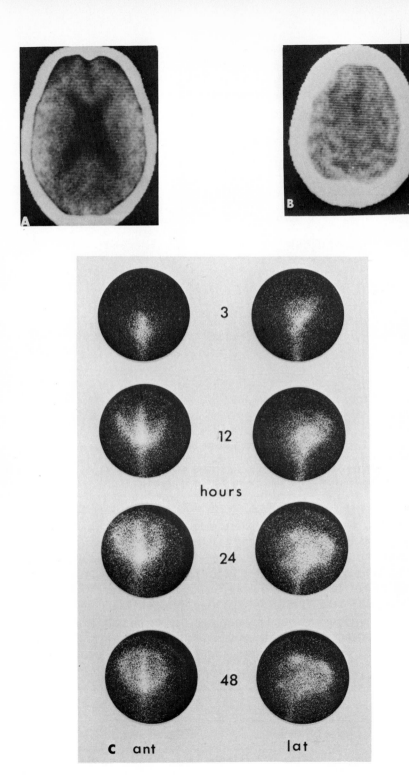

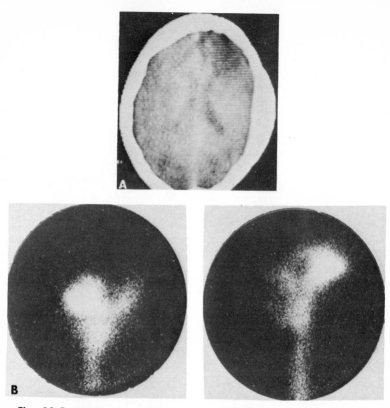

Fig. 11-5. ACTA scan and cisternogram of patient with porencephalic cyst. (A) ACTA scan shows cyst in right frontal lobe. Ventricular shift toward lesion suggests porencephaly rather than tumor. (B) Anterior (left) and right lateral (right) cisternogram shows accumulation of activity in cyst at 6 hr after injection.

ventricles, we believe that cisternography may be deferred and the patient followed by ACTA scans. When significant ventricular dilation and/or manifestations of elevated cerebrospinal fluid pressure exist, cisternography should be performed. With communicating hydrocephalus, shunting is probably needed unless there are no clinical symptoms. In the absence of ventricular reflux and if evidence of intracranial mass lesion exists, contrast studies must be done to rule out noncommunicating hydrocephalus.

References

1. LEDLEY RS, DiCHIRO G, LUESSENHOP AJ, et al: Computerized transaxial x-ray tomography of the human body. *Science* 186: 207–212, 1974

2. SCHELLINGER D, AXELBAUM SP, TWIGG HL, et al: Computed total body tomography with the ACTA-scanner. In *Tomography,* Viamonte M, ed, Chicago, American College of Radiology: to be published

3. SCHELLINGER D, DICHIRO G, AXELBAUM SP, et al: Early clinical experience with the ACTA-scanner. *Radiology* 114: 257–261, 1975

4. DICHIRO G, AXELBAUM SP, SCHELLINGER D, et al: Computerized axial tomography in syringomyelia. *N Engl J Med* 292: 13–16, 1975

5. PAXTON R, AMBROSE J: The EMI scanner. A brief review of the first 650 patients. *Br J Radiol* 47: 530–565, 1974

6. SCOTT WR, NEW PFJ, DAVIS KR, et al: Computerized axial tomography of intracerebral and intraventricular hemorrhage. *Radiology* 112: 73–80, 1974

7. BURROWS EH: False negative results in brain scanning. *Br Med J* 5798: 473–476, 1972

8. GATES GF, DORE EK, TAPLIN GV: Interval brain scanning with sodium pertechnetate- ^{99m}Tc for tumor detection. *JAMA* 215: 851, 1971

9. SCHALL GL, QUINN JL: Diagnosis of central nervous system disease. In *Nuclear Medicine,* Blahd W, ed, McGraw-Hill, 1971, chap 11

10. BAKER HL, CAMPBELL JK, HOUSER DW, et al: Computer assisted tomography of the head. An early evaluation. *Mayo Clin Proc* 49: 17–27, 1974

11. GAWLER J, DuBOULAY GH, BULL JWD, et al: Computer assisted tomography (EMI-Scanner). Its place in investigation of suspected intracranial tumors. *Lancet* 2: 419–423, 1974

12. NEW PFJ, SCOTT WR, SCHNUR JA, et al: Computed tomography with the EMI scanner in the diagnosis of primary and metastatic intracranial neoplasms. *Radiology* 114: 75–87, 1975

Chapter **12**

The Past, Present, and Future of Noninvasive Brain Imaging: Panel Discussion

Moderator:
Paul B. Hoffer

Discussants:
Philip Braunstein, Thomas F. Budinger, Edward Coleman,
Ernest W. Fordham, John C. Harbert, David E. Kuhl,
William H. Oldendorf, Michael E. Phelps,
Henry N. Wagner, Michael J. Welch

It always starts out as great fun to be the moderator of a discussion panel at a scientific meeting. For the rather cheap price of taking a few pertinent notes, one gains the reward of being able to virtually monopolize the interrogation of the panelists.

However, as with cheap wine, the headaches begin soon after. It is usually the moderator's responsibility to make sure that the panelists' remarks are preserved for posterity. Invariably it turns out that someone has forgotten to start the tape recorder on time. Listening to the original tapes reveals that, perhaps in deference to the laws of privacy, the recording volume has been set at the "almost audible" level. Small wonder that when the first manuscript comes back from the transcriber, an hour of intense scientific discussion has been converted into complete gibberish. After the initial editorial cosmetics, it becomes obvious that subject A was so interesting that nobody

Panel Discussion | 195

really wanted to give it up, and it resurfaces periodically throughout the entire discussion. Furthermore, Dr. X answered Dr. Y's question in the middle of Dr. W's soliloquy, and nobody ever really did get around to answering poor Dr. Z's question. After more vigorous editing, rearranging, and removal of 120 "Ah's" and other expletives, the original manuscript is sent to each participant with brave hopes that he will not so completely rewrite his section that it turns out to be longer than the other commentaries.

I must thank our panelists for being extremely considerate. Virtually all of them made very few substantive changes in the commentaries. They tolerated a considerable amount of editorial rearrangement of their remarks. They all accepted the use of the expression CTT (computerized transaxial tomography) as a substitute for the ten or so different abbreviations that we used during the actual discussion to describe the procedure.

Having had the "unique" opportunity of reading the manuscript about ten times, I remain impressed with both the quality of discussion and the broadness of its scope. There is information here for the physician in general practice and the specialist. There is information for the hospital administrator and regional health planner. Last but not least, there are the seeds of at least four or five research projects waiting here for the clever medical researcher.

Finally, my sincere thanks to the panelists for their tolerance and constructive editing and my humble apologies to Dr. Eichman of Florida, whose question was never really answered and, at the stroke of the editor's pen, has been "lost to followup."

Discussion

Dr. Hoffer: Some of the presentations at this symposium, in particular the presentation regarding the transaxial tomography positron detection system developed at the Mallinckrodt Institute of Radiology, describe extremely sophisticated and expensive devices. Are these devices the clinical instrumentation of the future or are they strictly research tools that will be used to guide the development of somewhat less sophisticated, less expensive devices?

Dr. Phelps: The prototype positron emission transaxial tomograph (PETT) was built to evaluate the design considerations and imaging capabilities of annihilation coincidence detection in transaxial tomography. The success of this system led to the question of whether to build a small system for research or to build a large system suitable for clinical study. Our decision was to build PETT III (Fig. 7–16), which is a clinical system suited for the tomographic imaging of the human head and torso. This system is presently undergoing clinical evaluation at the Mallinckrodt Institute of Radiology. Our current studies are twofold. The first involves the development of radiopharmaceuticals and procedures employing PETT III and ^{68}Ga from the long-lived ^{68}Ge-^{68}Ga generator system. The second is concerned with the use of cyclotron-produced positron emitters (^{18}F, ^{11}C, ^{13}N, and ^{15}O) incorporated into physiological substrates to yield "functional" images of metabolic processes with PETT III. Currently, most clinical procedures in nuclear medicine are oriented to the use of low-energy monochromatic radionuclides due to the imaging characteristics of the scintillation camera and scanners. We feel the same relationship exists between positron emitters and the positron transaxial tomograph. The clinical usefulness of this system will depend on our clinical results and those of investigators at the Massachusetts General Hospital, University of California at Los Angeles, and others who may build this type of system.

Dr. Welch: In order for the transaxial tomographic positron detection unit to be clinically successful, the ^{68}Ge-^{68}Ga generator will have to be developed beyond its current state. It should be remembered that it is over 10 years since Gottschalk and Anger (1) first used ^{68}Ga for brain scanning. It is not a new radiopharmaceutical.

Dr. Hoffer: The computerized transaxial tomographic units (CTT), such as the EMI scanner, are very sensitive to patient motion. Any significant amount of patient motion seriously interferes with the technical quality of the scan. The radionuclide brain scan is not nearly so sensitive to patient motion. Today we have heard two presentations, one by Dr. Coleman and the other by Dr. Passalaqua, discussing the relative sensitivity of these two brain-imaging techniques for screening patients for neurological disease. Were examinations with excessive patient motion included in the studies or rejected as "technically inadequate"? If scans were rejected as "technically inadequate," is such exclusion scientifically legitimate?

Dr. Coleman: In our study, those cases with motion artifact were excluded. Different problems may be encountered in studying patients by CTT scanning. One of these problems is motion artifact, which is especially prominent in children. Another problem in infants of particularly small head size is that firm contact of the rubber bag against the head is difficult to obtain. Another infrequent problem is the patient whose head is too large to fit into the rubber bag. CTT scans were attempted in such cases but were technically unsatisfactory, and only the radionuclide brain scan was obtained. These cases are rare and were excluded from our study.

Dr. Braunstein: We also excluded technically unsatisfactory studies in the material that was presented. More cases were excluded because of a technically inadequate CTT scan than because of a technically inadequate radionuclide scan. There are other reasons than just patient motion that can make CTT scans technically difficult or impossible to perform. These problems include the presence of clips or metallic plates in the brain and skull or the presence of any other dense materials such as pantopaque in the head.

Dr. Fordham: At our institution, more than 10% of CTT scans show some motion artifact, but these render the study uninterpretable in only 3% of the cases. Unfortunately, it is often in the very group of patients in which the CTT scan tends to be suboptimal that it is clinically most important to determine if there is a lesion present in the brain.

Dr. Hoffer: I would like to ask Drs. Coleman and Braunstein to tell us the exact number of studies that were eliminated for technical reasons for each procedure and also to give us some more detailed information as to why these studies were deemed to be inadequate.

Dr. Coleman: We excluded no study on the basis of inadequate radionuclide imaging. I do not have an exact number, but I believe there were approximately ten patients with intracranial mass lesions who had CTT scans that were technically inadequate. A CTT study was attempted by introducing the patient into the apparatus. However, after it became obvious that the patient would not cooperate, the examination was terminated at that point. With experience and proper premedication, the number of technically inadequate CTT scans has decreased.

Dr. Braunstein: In our study, we eliminated 33 patients altogether for various reasons. At most, one patient was eliminated from the series due to inadequate radionuclide study. Perhaps as many as ten cases were eliminated because of inadequate CTT studies. Most of these inadequate studies were due to patient motion. Occasionally, in postoperative patients, metallic clips produced totally obscuring artifacts. In one case, the presence of pantopaque made the CTT scan uninterpretable.

Dr. Hoffer: Many investigators feel that a CTT scan is not adequate unless a contrast agent is used. Dr. Oldendorf, could you tell us something about the localization of contrast agents in abnormal brain tissue? Is the mechanism similar to that associated with the localization of radionuclide agents in such lesions? If so, what is the advantage of such a contrast CTT scan over the conventional radionuclide brain scan?

Dr. Oldendorf: If a small molecule such as renografin is given systemically, it will leave the blood and equilibrate with the extracellular fluid with a blood disappearance of about 30 sec (2). The widely held belief that the CTT scan with contrast material is looking at blood in the brain is therefore not justified. You do see blood, but, even in the very few minutes following intravenous injection of the contrast agent, there is considerable equilibration with the extracellular fluid space that may be associated with brain lesions. With the

CTT scan, you are seeing much the same blood-brain barrier defect (when a contrast agent is used) as you are seeing in the radionuclide brain scan. When you give a contrast agent for a CTT study, you are essentially doing a high-resolution brain scan.

Dr. Harbert: I am not certain I agree with Dr. Oldendorf. The three lesions that show up most strikingly with a contrast agent on the CTT scan are vascular meningiomas, arteriovenous malformations (which do not show up at all without contrast), and the vascular portion of cystic lesions.

Dr. Oldendorf: In the ^{99m}Tc-DTPA or EDTA scans, the radionuclide is acting primarily as an extracellular fluid space marker and has a distribution very similar to the renografin in a CTT scan. With ^{99m}Tc-pertechnetate, approximately 75% of the activity in the blood is bound to plasma, and only about 25% is free in solution. This applies, however, only to the activity remaining in the blood. There is constant diffusion of the unbound material into the extracellular fluid, resulting in a shift of bound to unbound material in the blood, and further diffusion into the extracellular fluid. As a result, within a few minutes, most of the activity is in the extracellular fluid, not blood (2). I still think the major difference between the two studies is the superior resolution and display system of the CTT scan.

Dr. Braunstein: In our study, the detection rate using the noncontrast CTT scan combined with the contrast CTT scan was not quite as good as the combination of the noncontrast CTT scan and the radionuclide brain scan. The use of contrast agent in the CTT scan introduces a certain known risk of allergic or anaphylactic reaction, which is not present with the radionuclide brain scan.

Dr. Hoffer: It sounds as if some of the panelists feel it is the tomographic aspect of the CTT scan that makes it so appealing when compared with the radionuclide brain scan. Computerized transaxial tomographic radionuclide imaging systems have been built in prototype form and have been used clinically. What is preventing these systems from becoming commercially available?

Dr. Kuhl: In our earlier work with radionuclide or emission computerized tomography, we demonstrated to our satisfaction the clear advantage of the method as applied to brain tumor detection and localization (3). Perhaps we failed to convince enough potential users that the additional information on tumor presence and localization was crucial in the management of patients referred for study. I suspect that if a marketing analysis had been made several years ago, it might have shown a limited demand for introduction of a novel but expensive radionuclide computerized tomographic instrument, which, at that time, lacked the performance characteristics and potential for new applications that are now possible. Manufacturers were unwilling to invest in the development of a commercial radionuclide computerized tomographic instrument then, but the situation should be different now. Very efficient prototypes of radionuclide computerized tomography devices have been introduced at this meeting, better reconstruction strategies have evolved, and, most important, new and significant tests of local function are now being proposed that cannot be performed without radionuclide computerized tomography. I certainly hope that developments such as these will finally encourage commercial companies to make the new instruments widely available.

Dr. Budinger: Dr. Kuhl introduced the concept of radionuclide transaxial tomography by simple superposition or back-projection tomographic methods (4). The original method had certain limitations that were apparent from the outset. It was a low-resolution system to begin with, and this was further blurred by the tomographic reconstruction technique used from 1963 to 1973. Dr. Kuhl originally attempted to use the device to better detect and delineate posterior fossa tumors. His earlier clinical work indicated that the detection rate was no better with this instrument than with conventional brain scanning. However, the delineation of tumor was better, and this was important information for the neurosurgeon. At that point in the development of radionuclide transaxial tomographic systems, there were both instrumentation and mathematical problems. In 1968, as a result of a paper by DeRosier and Klug (5), there was renewed effort in many fields for the clear three-dimensional delineation of densities and radionuclide distributions using the transaxial tomographic approach. At that time, flexible computer systems were just beginning to be interfaced with scintillation cameras and rectilinear scanners. It took a few years for all of the interface problems to be effectively resolved. From the mathematical point of view, the development of algorithms for transaxial tomography, which now seems a very simple task, did not seem so simple a number of years ago. For example, we at Donner Laboratories were forced by research budget limitations to wait until 1971 to implement, with small computers, the systems that we had simulated with larger computer systems in 1968. It was not until the equipment and mathematical problems were resolved that we were able to develop sufficient data in the research laboratory to get the medical community excited about the capabilities of these systems. In the meantime, the CTT units came along. All of the work to which I have referred was done quite separately from the EMI device.

Even in 1968, we had spectacular examples of what could be achieved with radionuclide transaxial tomography. What we needed was a few years of clinical trials to convince clinicians of the utility of these images.

Dr. Oldendorf: I have some comments about the commercial viability of these very complex systems, since I think this is a vital part of their future development. In 1961, I developed and described (6) a system very similar to the Hounsfield system currently used by EMI, and I approached all of the x-ray companies between 1961 and 1964, asking them if they would be interested in developing my system. None of the companies were interested in the system. They did not reject it on technical grounds; they rejected it because, from a commercial standpoint, they could not imagine a market for such a system, which was just to draw a radiographic section of a head and would obviously cost several hundred thousand dollars.

One very important technical advance occurred in the past decade that paved the way for the viability of the EMI machine. That event was the introduction of the very expensive scintillation cameras. Ten years ago, the concept of spending $100,000 for a scintillation camera device was unthinkable. Even the original Anger cameras, which sold for approximately $30,000, were considered to be extravagantly expensive. Once the background of spending $100,000 or more for a single instrument was created, spending $300,000 to $400,000 for a single instrument was no longer inconceivable. In this regard, it is interesting that the vast majority of orders that have been placed for EMI devices have been from the United States. Now that a background has been established for the purchase of machines in the $400,000 price range, it begins to sound possible that you could market a machine costing $600,000 to $800,000. The machine described by the Mallinckrodt group, due to its technical complexity, could conceivably fall into that price range (see Dr. Phelps' comment at the end of discussion). However, even the American medical economic "plum pudding" is not bottomless, and I wonder when the point will be reached when the medical economy will no longer be able to support the cost of these ever increasingly elaborate and expensive machines.

Dr. Hoffer: The debate comparing radionuclide brain imaging and CTT imaging has been an acrimonious one. This has at least in part been due to the fact that there are two separate medical specialty groups performing these two studies. Does the panel feel that the interests both of patients and the medical community would be better served by having a single physician or group of physicians supervising both examinations?

Dr. Wagner: I think that scientific advances are to some degree based on specialization. If one is too general, one never makes any advances. In the introduction of a new device, it is important that we have people working with it who know what they are doing. The acrimony comes from personal characteristics rather than anything that has to do with science. However, in terms of general clinical application, I think that the evils of territoriality far outweigh the advantages. I do not believe that technological advances should be the exclusive domain of one person or group of persons. Regarding the clinical application of the computerized transaxial tomographic units, such as the EMI scanner and its relationship to current radionuclide brain scanning, we should use the particular instrument appropriate to the patient's problem. If the patient has a probable stroke, abscess, or infection such as Herpes encephalitis, I would recommend a radionuclide brain scan initially and see what the result of the scan was before ordering further tests. If the patient has the problem of senile dementia, I would do the CTT study first, since the probability of the patient having cerebral atrophy or hydrocephalus would be high. If I felt that there were a high probability of a meningioma, I would do a radionuclide brain scan. If the patient had a probable metastatic lesion, I would do a radionuclide brain scan because it is cheaper and the cost of missing the lesion, in terms of its medical implications for the patient, is not great. If the patient had a probable glioma, I would do a CTT scan first. If the patient had a probable subdural hematoma, I would do a scan in conjunction with a radionuclide bloodflow study and possibly do a CTT scan subsequently, depending on the level of my clinical suspicion. If the patient had a pituitary tumor, I would do a skull x-ray. If the patient had a very high probability of having a glioma of some sort, I would not hesitate to do both studies (CTT and brain scan). The idea of comparing one instrument to another for the detection of all lesions is not appealing to me.

Dr. Coleman: I agree with Dr. Wagner. When we initiated our study to compare CTT scanning with radionuclide imaging, we wanted to define what the inital procedure for evaluating a patient with a neurological problem should be. We discovered, however, that you cannot look at lesion detectability alone. It is necessary to evaluate patients in terms of presenting signs and symptoms and how the results of the study affect the management of the patient. It is also necessary to evaluate the cost/benefit aspects of these procedures. We are now attempting to investigate some of these factors. At the moment, we only have information on lesion detectability, which is interesting although of somewhat limited value. Until the studies are actually performed to determine the efficacy and cost effectiveness of these procedures as related to presenting signs and symptoms, it is very difficult to say which procedure should be done first and which patients should have both procedures.

Dr. Fordham: In most large teaching hospitals, 2–3 days of the patient's time are required in order to have the various consultants, such as the neurosurgeon and the neurologist, see and evaluate the patient. Since the cost of hospitalization itself is so expensive, the additional cost of a radionuclide brain scan, for instance, done in conjunction with the CTT scan is really not that large in relationship to the patient's total hospitalization costs. This, of course, does not pertain to outpatient workups.

Dr. Hoffer: I drew the inference from Dr. Wagner's earlier statements that he would like to see all consultations for either CTT or radionuclide brain scans directed to a single consultant group or individual who would have particular expertise with regard to which study would be preferable and in what sequence the patient evaluation should be performed. Such a system sounds highly desirable to me and I wonder if the other panelists feel that this would be a reasonable and responsible approach.

Dr. Wagner: This is a reasonable approach, but it is not the one that I suggested. I personally would not follow that plan. In view of the increasing specialization in medicine, I would prefer a team approach. The best example is the approach to the cancer patient, which involves the combined efforts of the radiation therapist, chemotherapist, and surgeon. I do not know why we do not use the same approach for diagnostic problems as well. A model that comes to my mind is evaluation of a mass that is detected on chest x-ray. I believe that the evaluation of such a lesion should be a joint diagnostic effort on the part of the cytologist, bronchoscopist, radiologist, and pathologist. I believe that people who try to take everything under their own wing are not going to prevail; they will continue to have trouble from people who do not like territoriality.

Serious consideration should be given to the question of whether the patient with neurological problems should receive a routine workup versus a flexible workup tailor-made to the patient's problem. In some situations, it is probably preferable to do things on a routine basis. However, we continue to labor under the problem of how much to tailor-make our radionuclide tracer studies to our patient's problems. When we try to tailor-make the study, it becomes very expensive. We require a doctor to examine the patient prior to the study and determine whether the patient should, for instance, have a bloodflow study or posterior fossa views. This is not an efficient approach from a mass production viewpoint. I am still personally struggling with the problem of what should be routine in the nuclear medicine department and what should be tailor-made, depending on the patient's problem.

Dr. Harbert: I recently had the opportunity to work with the regional health care groups from the city of Denver, helping them determine how many instruments of the transaxial tomographic (CTT) type should be adequate for that geographic area. Every regional health care organization is going to be faced with this type of decision in the near future, and therefore it becomes imperative that we define which is going to be the appropriate screening test for patients with nonspecific or "soft" neurologic signs and symptoms such as headache, seizures, ill-defined sensory changes, paresthesias, and the like. While we would like to believe that radionuclide brain scanning and transaxial tomography augment one another, I believe that the lion's share of the screening is going to fall to the computerized tomographic devices because they have much broader utility in the evaluation of neurological disease, as well as better accuracy.

Dr. Braunstein: I would like to defend at least the occasional use of the combined computerized transverse tomographic study and the radionuclide brain scan from the point of view of cost. In patients with a relatively high index of suspicion for having a brain lesion, the clinician in the presence of a negative CTT or radionuclide brain scan will go on to an angiographic study. However, it has been our experience that if the CTT scan and the radionuclide brain scan are negative, the clinician will not then proceed to an angiographic study. The saving of an unnecessary angiographic procedure certainly to some extent compensates for the cost of doing the combined studies in some patients.

Dr. Wagner: I would like to ask Dr. Harbert a question that worries me. We all agree that one of the most important functions of all of these studies is to decrease the likelihood that a patient has a serious disease. The radionuclide brain scan is particularly sensitive to detection of meningioma, which is by far the most important brain tumor to diagnose. If it turns out that the CTT scan without contrast is not highly sensitive for detection of meningioma, do you anticipate that contrast agents will be used as a routine screening procedure in patients who are suspected of having brain tumors?

Dr. Harbert: I suspect that for the detection of meningiomas we will probably rely on CTT imaging. Paxton and Ambrose, reporting in the *British Journal of Radiology* (7), detected 34 of 35 patients with meningiomas for a 97% accuracy. Dr. Baker's group at Mayo Clinic detected 21 of 23 cases for an accuracy of 91% (8), and New and colleagues recently reported detection of 11 of 11 cases for 100% accuracy (9).

Dr. Wagner: Are those results obtained with or without contrast agents?

Dr. Harbert: Most of those results were obtained with the use of contrast agents.

Dr. Hoffer: Dr. New's studies, in which he detected 11 of 11 meningiomas, were performed without the use of contrast agents.

Dr. Wagner: Conflicting reports about whether or not contrast medium is necessary are what causes confusion. A procedure is introduced (such as the use of a contrast agent with CTT imaging) and yet the procedure that it is replacing is already believed to be perfect. Last year's test was perfect, and this year's test is even better. It becomes impossible to say from the published results whether or not you really need a contrast agent in order to detect meningioma with a greater than 95% probability.

Dr. Hoffer: What new noninvasive methods are being developed for diagnosis of brain pathology and what improvements do the panelists foresee in CTT imaging or conventional radionuclide brain scanning?

Dr. Oldendorf: In addition to the rather elaborate systems discussed here today, there is at least one method that I believe can be applied to improve brain scanning that could probably be done by many of the people here. The method would be to perform brain scan images in which you would subtract the extracranial contribution. I have been trying to get somebody to do this since 1969. I am a clinical neurologist with no direct contact with clinical nuclear medicine and have not had an opportunity to implement this technique myself. Above the floor of the cranial cavity, 90% of the activity seen on the normal brain scan is contributed by radionuclide localized in the scalp and the skull. This activity contributes only to the general background surrounding the brain, and it obscures the underlying regional differences in activity that we want to see. Therefore, it could well be useful to try to develop methods that would eliminate this extracranial activity, especially in the posterior fossa, which is frequently badly obscured. The method I proposed some years ago (*10*) is to use the characteristic x-ray output of some of the commonly used radionuclides to quantitate the superficial component of the activity. The characteristic x-ray output occurs in a fixed ratio to the gamma output; you can, for example, with ^{99m}Tc take the 18-keV x-ray, which occurs in a ratio of about one x-ray to 15 gammas. One would window on the gamma output and separately window on the x-ray, treating it as if it were a second isotope. Using this system, 15 gammas would be subtracted for every x-ray seen. This would subtract a number of gammas equal to those that are being emitted extracranially. In this way, you could correct at least for the extracranial components of activity from the scalp. This system would work better with ^{113m}In, which has a 24-keV x-ray, which occurs in a ratio of 1:3 with the gamma emission.

Dr. Budinger: There is no excuse for not having an image on line immediately after a scan procedure is performed. Electronically, this is simple to do with hard-wired algorithms, which certainly will be a future development.

It is quite easy to get an image of the ventricles using the Toshiba transverse axial tomographic unit, which is a film unit not utilizing a computer. An area of development will be to improve the quality and availability of such units, which are able to demonstrate 10% differences in attenuation rather than the 2% or 3% differences for which the computerized tomographic devices are required. These noncomputerized units could be used to look at grosser structures.

I would also like to ask a question of the panel. Why is it not possible to use xenon dissolved in saline as a noninvasive technique for looking at permeability with the EMI scanner?

Dr. Welch: In order to perform such a study, it would be necessary to have a great deal of xenon dissolved in a small amount of saline. I do not see any way that you could possibly get enough into solution.

Dr. Phelps: I believe that the amount of xenon that you would have to give would be an anesthetic dose rather than a tracer dose.

Dr. Hoffer: There have been studies performed using fluorescent techniques which indicate that, if inhalation techniques are used, rather large amounts of xenon can be localized in the brain tissue. Xenon is a relatively expensive gas when high purity is required. However, for administration of xenon by inhalation, high purity is not required, and with the use of rebreathing apparatus, the cost of the xenon can be reduced to a conceivable, if not practical, figure.

Dr. Kuhl: Xenon is a freely diffusible indicator. I would think it a poor choice for measuring changes in blood-brain barrier. Would not a less diffusible indicator be preferred?

Dr. Hoffer: This, of course, depends on what you are looking for. Some empiricists feel that if you have a material that is freely diffusible in the brain and highly fat soluble and can be used as a contrast agent for CTT imaging, why not go ahead and use it and see what it shows.

Dr. Hirsch Handmaker (Children's Hospital, San Francisco, Calif.): What is the charge at the panelist's institutions for a radionuclide brain scan? What is the charge for a CTT scan? Is there a recharge if the CTT study is repeated using contrast material and why is contrast material not used routinely since it seems to improve the detection rate with the CTT scan?

Dr. Coleman: Our charge is $105 for the brain scan and $25 for the radionuclide angiogram. The charge for the CTT scan is $230. All CTT scans are done initially without contrast. Repeat scans with contrast are done in two groups of patients: (A) those who have normal scans and a high probability of having a lesion based on history and physical examination, and (B) those who have an initially abnormal CTT, for better delineation of the lesion. No additional charge is made for the contrast study.

Dr. Braunstein: The charge for our radionuclide brain scan is about $150. The charge for the EMI (CTT) scan is about $240. Approximately 50% of the patients studied with the CTT scan are repeated with contrast. Our neuroradiology group does not routinely use contrast initially since they have seen cases in which the lesion was originally lucent or less dense than the surrounding brain and actually disappeared following the administration of a contrast agent. They are concerned that they might miss lesions if they just did contrast studies.

Dr. Hoffer: At the University of California, San Francisco, the charge for a radionuclide brain scan is $107. The charge for the CTT scan is $200 without contrast agent and about $250 with contrast agent.

What about new radiopharmaceuticals for brain imaging?

Dr. Budinger: Rubidium-82 can be extracted from an [82]Sr generator. This radionuclide has been investigated by Yano. It is a positron emitter and can be used with the positron-type transverse axial tomographic radionuclide devices. We have also been investigating its use in the single gamma mode. It has promise for measurement of cerebral blood flow.

Dr. Welch: The sort of thing that I can foresee is the use of other rare gases. Dr. DeNardo and associates (University of California, Davis) have developed other rare gases to replace [133]Xe. The group at Brookhaven National Laboratory is working on the production of a bromine-selenium generator to produce a very short-lived radionuclide. Another approach that I think may be highly successful for answering the need for a highly lipid-soluble ^{99m}Tc-labeled tracer would be the use of a double-end chelate, such as those being developed by Dr. David Goodwin of Stanford University to label ^{99m}Tc to a highly fat-soluble substrate.

Dr. Kuhl: Hoffer and associates (*11*) have suggested the replacement of ^{133}Xe by [127]Xe because of its superior physical characteristics. I understand that [127]Xe will soon be available from the Brookhaven National Laboratory.

Dr. Z.H. Cho (University of California, Los Angeles): Is it fair to compare the images that are produced with the CTT unit, which has an extremely elaborate display system, with the images produced on a conventional radionuclide imaging device, which has a significantly less elaborate display system?

Dr. Phelps: In answer to Dr. Cho's question, it may be unfair to compare the transmission and emission transaxial tomographs to the conventional system from an instrumentation point of view, but the real question that must be answered is whether these new systems provide an improvement in diagnostic evaluation and prognosis for the patient.

Earlier in this discussion, the question arose regarding the equipment cost of the positron tomographic units. Our system is complex, although not as complex as it appears to be. However, any transaxial tomograph is going to be more complex than, say, a stationary scintillation camera or radiographic unit. It is not easy for a research group to determine what the ultimate cost of a product would be. It is sometimes difficult for us to appreciate and evaluate all the costs that go into commercial production, distribution, and support of a new instrument. However, I do not agree with Dr. Oldendorf that the system will cost anywhere near the figure that he has given.

References

1. ANGER HO, GOTTSCHALK A: Localization of brain tumors with the positron scintillation camera. *J Nucl Med* 4: 326–330, 1963

2. OLDENDORF WH: Distribution of various classes of radiolabeled tracers in plasma, scalp, and brain. *J Nucl Med* 13: 681–685, 1972

3. KUHL DE, SANDERS TP: Characterizing brain lesions using transverse section scanning. *Radiology* 98: 317–328, 1971

4. KUHL DE, EDWARDS RQ: Image separation radioisotope scanning. *Radiology* 80: 653–662, 1963

5. DeROSIER DJ, KLUG A: Reconstruction of three-dimensional structures from electron micrographs. *Nature* (Lond) 217: 130–134, 1968

6. OLDENDORF WH: Isolated flying spot detection of radiodensity discontinuities—displaying the internal structural pattern of a complex object. *Inst Radio Eng Trans Biomed Electron* 8: 68–72, 1961

7. PAXTON R, AMBROSE J: The EMI scanner. A brief review of the first 650 patients. *Br J Radiol* 47: 530–565, 1974

8. BAKER HL, CAMPBELL JK, HOUSER DW, et al: Computer assisted tomography of the head. An early evaluation. *Mayo Clin Proc* 49: 17–27, 1974

9. NEW PFJ, SCOTT WR, SCHNUR J A, et al: Computed tomography with the EMI scanner in the diagnosis of primary and metastatic intracranial neoplasms. *Radiology* 114: 75–87, 1975

10. OLDENDORF WH: Utilization of characteristic x-radiation to identify gamma radiation originating external to the skull. *J Nucl Med* 10: 740–742, 1969

11. HOFFER PB, HARPER PV, BECK RN, et al: Improved xenon images with xenon-127. *J Nucl Med* 14: 172–174, 1973

Index

Attenuation correction
   positron emission transaxial tomograph, 97–98
   static three-dimensional camera imaging, 60–63
Automatic computerized transverse axial scanner (see ACTA scanner, scanning)

B

Back projection reconstruction techniques
   in CTT, 118–119, 121–123
   linear superposition, 118–119, 121–123
   panel discussion, 200
   static three-dimensional camera imaging, 59
Benzylamine (see Carbon-11-benzylamine)
Bicarbonate (see Carbon-11-bicarbonate)
Blood
   attenuation coefficient, 126
   hematocrit (see Hematocrit)
   pH (see pH, blood)
Blood-brain barrier penetration, 17–23, 31, 34–37
   ^{11}C-alcohols, 31, 34–37
   capillary characteristics, 17–19
   carrier-mediated, 19–23
   endothelial cells, 18
   experimental studies (in rats), 19–20
   extracellular fluid, 18
   lipid-mediated, 19–23
   molecular criteria, 17–23
   nonpolar drugs, 19
   pinocytosis, 18
   polar solutes, 19
   radiolabeled water, 34
   ^{75}Se-selenomethionine, 21
Blood clot
   attenuation coefficient, 126
   radionuclide imaging and CTT, comparisons, 161
Blood flow
   computer analysis, 4–6, 45–51
   ^{123}I-iodoantipyrine, limitations, 21
   ^{131}I-iodoantipyrine, 20–21
   inert gases, 30–31
   lipid-soluble tracers, gaseous vs. nonvolatile, 21
   ^{15}O-water studies, 27–28
   radionuclide study, for subdural hematoma, panel discussion, 202

^{82}Rb, panel discussion, 207
   serial imaging, 4–6
   ^{99m}Tc compounds, 21
   ^{99m}Tc-pertechnetate, 47
   xenon, 21
Blood plasma, attenuation coefficient, 126
Blood volume
   CRTT (Mark III) scanning, 70–77
   equilibrium imaging, 53–54
   ^{15}O-labeled radiopharmaceuticals, 28–29, 40–41
   static three-dimensional camera imaging, 55–64
Brain (see specific subject)
Brain floor lesions, ACTA and radionuclide scans, comparison, 188
Brain stem
   glioma, ACTA and radionuclide scans, comparison, 188
   pertechnetate scanning, relative accuracy, 15
Brain tissue, attenuation coefficients, 126
Brain tumors (see the specific disease, procedure, or site)
Bromine-selenium generator, for short-lived radionuclides, panel discussion, 207
Butanol (see Carbon-11-butanol)
Butyrate, blood-brain barrier penetration, 22

C

Calvarial lesions, Anger tomoscanner, 81–86
Cameras (see Scintillation cameras)
Capillaries, blood-brain barrier, characteristics, 17–19
Carbon-11
   central nervous system studies, 31–40
   cerebral hematocrit measurement, 37–40
   equilibrium imaging, 41
   intracellular pH determinations, 41
   PETT scan, in dogs, 101–105
   PETT III scans, panel discussion, 197
   production, 31
   psychotropic drugs
      cerebral uptake studies, 42
      tomographic possibilities, 42
Carbon-11-acetoacetate, metabolism studies, 31

Carbon-11-acetoacetic acid
  ketogenic substrate metabolism, 33
  production, 33–34
Carbon-11-albumin
  cerebral hematocrit measurement, 37–40
  production, 37–38
Carbon-11-alcohols, blood-brain barrier permeability studies, 31, 34–37
Carbon-11-amines, equilibrium imaging, in estimating intracellular pH, 41
Carbon-11-benzylamine, equilibrium imaging, in estimation of intracellular pH, 41
Carbon-11-bicarbonate, pH studies, 31–32
Carbon-11-butanol, blood-brain barrier permeability studies, 35–36
Carbon-11-glucose
  metabolism studies, 31–34
  PETT III scan, 103
  production, 32–33
Carbon-11-hemoglobin, PETT III scan, 104–107
Carbon-11-labeled psychotropic drugs
  cerebral uptake studies, 42
  tomographic possibilities, 42
Carbon-11-methanol, blood-brain barrier permeability studies, 34–37
Carbon-11-methyl albumin, hematocrit measurement, 37–40
Carbon-11-nicotine, equilibrium imaging, in estimation of intracellular pH, 41–42
Carbon-11-pentylamine, equilibrium imaging, in estimating intracellular pH, 41
Carbon-11-proteins, and cerebral hematocrit studies, 31
Carbon-11-quinine, equilibrium imaging, in estimating intracellular pH, 41
Carbon-14-imipramine, regional blood flow study, 21
Carboxyhemoglobin (see Oxygen-15-carboxyhemoglobin)
Carotid occlusion
  blood flow, counts vs. time calculations, 48–49
  T-MAX vertex image, 53
Carotid stenosis, blood flow, counts vs. time calculations, 48–49
Central nervous system (see specific subject)
Cerebellopontine angle, pertechnetate

scanning, relative accuracy, 9, 10, 15
Cerebellum, pertechnetate scanning, relative accuracy, 9
Cerebral studies (see specific subject)
Cerebrospinal fluid
  attenuation coefficient, 126
  radionuclide cisternography and CTT scanning, comparisons, 162–168
Cerebrovascular disease
  pertechnetate scanning, relative efficacy, 14, 15
  radionuclide imaging and CTT scanning, comparisons, 158–162, 175, 178–179
Chloroma, ACTA scan and radionuclide imaging, comparison, 185
Cholesteoma, fourth ventricle, radionuclide cisternography and CTT, clinical comparisons, 175, 176
Cisternography
  and ACTA scanning, comparisons, 189–192
  and CTT, comparisons, 162–168, 175
Coincidence detection of positron-emitting radionuclides (see also, PETT scanner), 87–109
Collimators
  annihilation coincidence detection, 90
  multiprobe, for studying ^{15}O-labeled tracers, 27
  parallel hole, in static three-dimensional camera imaging, 58
  pinhole, in static three-dimensional camera imaging, 55
Compton scattering, 125–126, 133, 135
Computerized radionuclide transaxial tomography (see CRTT)
Computerized transaxial transmission tomography (see CTT)
Contrast
  CTT scanning, 136–138
  PETT scanner, 92–93
Contrast agents, panel discussion, 198–199, 204–205
Convolution algorithm, in transaxial transmission tomography, 133
Copper-64
  annihilation coincidence detection, 90–91, 94, 100–101
  cold spot reconstruction, PETT, 100–101
  spatial resolution, PETT, 98–101
Craniopharyngioma

spatial variation in attenuation coefficients, 136
statistical quality of image, 127–128, 134–135, 138
water, EMI value, 137
water box, 130–134, 188–189
x-ray tube potential, 130
"Cupping and capping" artifact, ACTA scans, 188–189
Cyclotron-produced positron emitters, for CNS studies, panel discussion, 197
Cysts
  porencephalic, radionuclide cisternography and ACTA scan, comparison, 190, 192
  radionuclide imaging and CTT, clinical comparisons, 148–158, 175–176

D

Defocusing effect, in CTT scanning, 118
Detector systems
  CRTT scanner
    Mark III scanner, 68
    Mark IV scanner, 77
  CTT scanner, 114, 142–143
  PETT scanner, 90, 91, 95–98
DTPA (see Indium-111-DTPA; Technetium-99m-DTPA; Ytterbium-169-DTPA)
Durovascular malformation, radionuclide imaging and CTT scan, comparison, 155
Dynamic time-dependent analysis, 45–51
  benefits, 50–51
  counts vs. time curves, 47–51
  derived quantitative parameters, 50–51
  integration of counts to first maximum, 47
  quantitation, background and fundamental problems, 45–47
  transit time calculation, 47
  uptake slope and time-to-peak activity, 47

E

Edematous tissue, attenuation coefficient, 126
EDTA (see Gallium-68-EDTA; Technetium-99m-EDTA)
Electroencephalography, relative accuracy, 5–10

EMI scanner (see also, CTT scanning)
  and ACTA scanner, comparison, 184, 188–189
  basic principles, 114–115
  cost, panel discussion, 201
  in clinical comparisons of radionuclide imaging and CTT, 147–171, 173–181
  motion artifact, 142
  motion artifact, panel discussion, 197
  reconstruction algorithms, 116–117
  values for different types of plastics, 134–135
  values for water, 137
Emission transaxial scanning (see CRTT scanning)
Encephalitis, herpes, diagnostic procedure, panel discussion, 202
Endothelial cells, blood-brain barrier, 18
Ependymoma, pertechnetate scanning, relative accuracy, 8
Equilibrium imaging
  definition, 53–54
  ^{15}O-labeled tracers, 40–41, 54
  short-lived radiopharmaceuticals, 40–42
Extracellular fluid, in blood-brain barrier penetration, 18

F

Fat, subcutaneous, attenuation coefficients, 126
"Flip-flop" phenomenon, T-MAX image, 52
Fluorescent techniques, panel discussion, 206
Fluorine-18
  glucose analogs, for glucose metabolism studies, 33–34
  PETT III scans, panel discussion, 197
Fourier-based reconstruction algorithm
Fresnel zone plate imaging, 56–58
  in CTT, 121–123, 134, 141–142
  in static three-dimensional camera imaging, 58–59
  PETT scanner, 97
Fresnel zone plate images, digital reconstruction, 56–58
Frontal tumors, pertechnetate scanning, relative accuracy, 6, 9
Frontoparietal tumors, pertechnetate scanning, relative accuracy, 9
D-Fructose, blood-brain barrier penetration, 22
Functional imaging, 52–54

G

Galactose, blood-brain barrier penetration, 21

Gallium-68
  ^{68}Ge-^{68}Ga generator system, panel discussion, 197
  PETT scanning, future potential, 106

Germanium-68
  ^{68}Ga generator system, panel discussion, 197

Glioblastoma multiforme, radionuclide imaging and CTT, comparisons, 152–153

Glioma
  brainstem, ACTA and radionuclide scans, comparison, 188
  diagnostic procedure, panel discussion, 202
  malignant
    blood volume studies, 76
    CRTT (Mark III) scan, 76
    pertechnetate scan, 76
  optic, pertechnetate scanning, relative accuracy, 8
  radionuclide imaging and CTT, comparisons, 148–158, 175, 176
  thalamus, ACTA and radionuclide scans, comparison, 188

Glucose (see also, Carbon-11-glucose)
  blood-brain barrier penetration, 21–22
  metabolism, ^{18}F-labeled glucose analogs, 33–34

H

Hamartoma, radionuclide imaging and CTT, comparison, 175

Hard-wired reconstruction algorithms, panel discussion, 205

Head size, problems, in transaxial tomography, panel discussion, 197

Hemangioblastoma, ACTA and radionuclide scans, comparison, 185

Hematocrit, cerebral
  ^{11}C-labeled tracers, 37–40
  ^{11}C-protein studies, 31
  equilibrium imaging, 40–41
  ^{15}O-labeled tracers, 40–41

Hematoma
  intracerebral
    CRTT (Mark III) and CTT scans, comparison, 70–71
    pertechnetate scan, 71

radionuclide imaging and ACTA scan, comparisons, 184–188
radionuclide imaging and CTT, comparisons, 161–162
subdural
  attenuation coefficient, 126
  blood flow, counts vs. time calculations, 48–49
  diagnostic procedure, panel discussion, 202
  radionuclide imaging and ACTA scan, comparisons, 185–187
  radionuclide imaging and CTT, comparisons, 148–158, 175, 179
  thalamus, radionuclide imaging and ACTA scan, comparisons, 186

Hemoglobin (see Carbon-11-hemoglobin)

Hemorrhage, intracerebral, radionuclide imaging and CTT, comparisons, 178

Hexoses, blood-brain barrier transport, 21–22

Hydrocephalus
  diagnostic procedure, panel discussion, 202
  radionuclide cisternography
    and ACTA scans, comparisons, 189–192
    and CTT, comparisons, 162–168, 175

β-Hydroxybutyrate, blood-brain barrier penetration, 22

I

Imipramine (see Carbon-14-imipramine)

Indium-111-DTPA
  cerebrospinal fluid cisternography, comparison to CTT, 162–168
  hydrocephalus, cisternography, and ACTA scan, comparisons, 189–192

Inert gas radionuclides
  blood flow studies, 30–31
  characteristics, 31

Infarction
  brainstem, radionuclide imaging and CTT, comparisons, 178
  cerebral
    blood flow, counts vs. time calculations, 48–49
    radionuclide imaging and ACTA scan, comparisons, 185
    radionuclide imaging and CTT, comparisons, 70, 72–73, 158–162, 178–179
    scintillation camera study, 73